STUDY GUIDE
FOR
FUNDAMENTALS
OF ANATOMY & PHYSIOLOGY,
Second Edition

BY
DONALD C. RIZZO, Ph.D.

Prepared By
Carolee G. Jones, Ph.D.

and

Ronald F. Jones

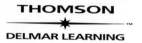

THOMSON

DELMAR LEARNING

Study Guide for Fundamentals of Anatomy & Physiology, Second Edition
by Donald C. Rizzo

Vice President, Health Care Business Unit:
William Brottmiller

Editorial Director:
Cathy L. Esperti

Acquisitions Editor:
Marah Bellegarde

Developmental Editor:
Debra Flis

Editorial Assistant:
Jadin Babin-Kavanaugh

Marketing Director:
Jennifer McAvey

Marketing Channel Manager:
Tamara Caruso

Marketing Coordinator:
Michele Gleason

Production Director:
Carolyn Miller

Production Manager:
Barbara A. Bullock

Art and Design Coordinator:
Alexandros Vasilakos

Production Coordinator:
Jessica McNavich

Project Editor:
Ruth Fisher

ISBN 1-4018-7189-5

NOTICE TO THE READER

Publisher does not warrant or guarantee any of the products described herein or perform any independent analysis in connection with any of the product information contained herein. Publisher does not assume, and expressly disclaims, any obligation to obtain and include information other than that provided to it by the manufacturer.

The reader is expressly warned to consider and adopt all safety precautions that might be indicated by the activities described herein and to avoid all potential hazards. By following the instructions contained herein, the reader willingly assumes all risks in connection with such instructions.

The publisher makes no representations or warranties of any kind, including but not limited to, the warranties of fitness for particular purpose or merchantability, nor are any such representations implied with respect to the material set forth herein, and the publisher takes no responsibility with respect to such material. The publisher shall not be liable for any special, consequential, or exemplary damages resulting, in whole or part, from the reader's use of, or reliance upon, this material.

TABLE OF CONTENTS

TO THE LEARNER

You have chosen a career in some aspect of the health care field. By so doing you have accepted the responsibility for gaining knowledge of the human body's structure and how it functions. This means learning the language associated with anatomy and physiology. Your text and this workbook were written to help you gain a basic knowledge of anatomy and physiology and their terminology. The text supplies the necessary information. This study guide will help you review and reinforce that knowledge.

ORGANIZATION OF THE STUDY GUIDE

Each chapter in the study guide corresponds to the same chapter in the text. The activities in each chapter follow the sequence of information presented in the text. A variety of questions and exercises are included to help reinforce the material you have learned in different ways. Types of activities in each chapter include completion, matching, key terms, labeling exercises, coloring exercises, critical thinking questions and crossword puzzles. Each chapter begins with the statement of chapter objectives. A quiz at the end of each chapter is designed to help you measure your grasp of those objectives.

As you proceed through each chapter of the text, complete the activities provided in this study guide to reinforce the material presented in class.

The following steps are recommended for using this book:

1. Read the chapter objectives.
2. Study the material presented in the text.
3. Listen carefully to the instructor.
4. Take comprehensive notes.
5. Ask questions.
6. Complete and correct the activities in the study guide.
7. Complete and correct the chapter quizzes in the study guide.
8. Review those concepts missed.

This study guide was prepared as a tool to help you learn. The author hopes this tool will help you gain the knowledge of anatomy and physiology necessary for success in your chosen career.

Thomas W. Owen, MS, CMA

STUDY TIPS AND TEST-TAKING STRATEGIES

STUDY AIDS TO HELP ENHANCE LEARNING

Learning is a process, the process of expanding your knowledge in a proportional manner. Each new piece of knowledge you gain allows you to expand your mind proportionally. How much information have you acquired since learning to read? The learning process ends only with the cessation of life.

Some learners feel overwhelmed at the beginning of a course because of the size of a text and the huge amount of information it contains. Yet, the longest journey begins with the first step. Each word, sentence, paragraph and chapter helps you learn that which follows. You have taken the first step on your journey to learn about the human body. As you continue that journey, you will become aware of your own anatomy and how your body functions. Use that awareness to build on your knowledge. You carry a "cheat sheet" (your body) everywhere you go. Use it to help you learn.

Reading

It is important to read the text more than once. It is also important that the material be read before it is covered in class. Read the chapter through in its entirety. Reread the chapter section by section. You will note that section headings indicate the nature of the material to be covered and highlight important points or concepts. Note that definitions, explanations and other emphasized material are usually in bold print. Make notes in the margins, including any questions you might have for your instructor. Sometimes difficult sections can be more easily understood by rewriting the passages in your own words. This helps identify where your problem is in understanding the chapter. After the material has been covered in class, read it again. It is important to note any concepts you do not understand so you may discuss them with the instructor.

The environment in which you read has a great deal of effect on how well you absorb and assimilate the material. A warm room and a comfortable chair are fine for reading a novel or the Sunday comics; however, when reading or studying textual material, it is best to be in a cool room (not uncomfortably cold) sitting up at a desk or table with good lighting. Reading after a hearty meal tends to make one sleepy and negatively affects concentration. Try to limit outside distractions such as television. Pick a time when such distractions are absent or at a minimum. Next, make a short outline using the section headings. Make this outline succinct and use one page for each heading. This is in preparation for note taking that is discussed next.

Listening and Taking Notes

You have read and reread the material for the upcoming class and made appropriate highlights and notations. Now you are ready for the next step in the learning process—listening to the instructor as he or she makes the presentation.

Most of us have little or no formal training in listening skills. There is more to listening than just being quiet and paying attention. During a presentation, it is advisable to take good comprehensive notes. How does one hear, process, write and comprehend all at once? By reading the material beforehand, making notations, highlighting and making an outline, the learner has a format with which to work. Good instructors will usually present along the lines of the chapter outline. They will use a lead sentence explaining what is to come next. They will emphasize important points, explain the material and sum up with a review at the conclusion of the lecture. After each segment of material, they will solicit questions for anyone needing further clarification. Be sure to ask questions if you need help understanding. Remember, the only dumb questions are those not asked. Using an outline will make it easier to listen attentively, process what is heard and make notes or jot questions as the presentation progresses.

Listening correctly takes effort and concentration. This means leaving personal problems at the classroom door. It means sitting erect and focusing on the instructor, not on fellow students or the view outside the classroom window. Come to class well prepared, having read and reread the material, highlighted, made notations and outlined; being well rested and having the necessary materials at hand. All this will ensure you are making the best possible effort to absorb and assimilate the material to be learned. After class, you will want to review your notes and compare them with the text to maximize understanding and reinforce learning.

Plan Your Studying

Most people plan their daily activities from rising in the morning to retiring in the evening. When studying it is also wise to plan. Preparation of the proper materials and avoidance of distractions are a necessity for the formation of good study habits.

Your place of study should be in a room that is not too warm (inducing sleepiness) and not too cool (inducing discomfort). Lighting should be adequate or your eyes will become strained, resulting in distraction. Do not get too comfortable in an easy chair; instead sit erect at a desk or table. Choose a time when family members are asleep, away or busy elsewhere. Although some people find music a distraction, others find it helps concentration (if not too loud). Television, on the other hand, is always a distraction. Studying after a heavy meal is a sure way to fall asleep, yet a totally empty stomach will clamor for attention, forcing concentration on food rather than study material. Keep the necessary materials in one place. Having to round up the tools for studying before each session is not conducive to a productive session. One helpful strategy may be to place yourself on an "if . . . then" contingency. For example, if you read Chapter 3, then you can go to dinner or a movie or some other reward that will work for you.

Group Studying

There are pros and cons to group study sessions. Having the ability to exchange ideas, clarify concepts through discussion and test one another's grasp of the material is often helpful. However, it is advisable to know each group member well enough so that digression and other distractions do not become part of the session. Proper environment, good preparation and no distractions are a must if the sessions are to be worthwhile.

Workbook Activities and Review

You have read the chapter objectives, chapter outline and the chapter material. You have read the chapter section by section and made the appropriate notations. You made an outline, listened well, asked questions, took notes and reviewed the material after class. How can you enhance your grasp of the chapter objectives further? Another step in the learning process is the completion of your workbook activities. They are designed to aid you in retention and reinforcement of the textual material. After you have completed the activities, taken the end-of-chapter test and corrected all your work, you will have a good idea of how much of the material you have learned. Do not stop there. Do not feel that once you have mastered a chapter you can move on without a backward glance. The text is organized to build on previously learned material. However, it is not possible to do this 100% of the time. Go back and review earlier chapters on a regular basis. Use your new-found knowledge every day if possible. The more you learn and use what you have learned, the more enjoyable the learning process will be.

Using the Internet as a Resource

The Internet provides access to valuable information about the body and anything that relates to health issues. Three sites in particular serve as a gateway to a plethora of information. They are:

National Institutes of Health http://www.nih.gov

United States National Library of Medicine http://www.nlm.nih.gov

Medline Plus, a service of the National Library of Medicine and the National Institutes of Health http://www.nlm.nih.gov (Click on the Medline Plus icon.)

These sites contain links to many other sources of information and should be used whenever you would like to expand your knowledge of a concept or process related to the health field.

HELPFUL HINTS FOR TAKING TESTS

There are highly intelligent, extremely well-prepared learners who experience test anxiety to the point of having brain freeze on test day. In reality we are tested every day. A test is a tool to measure what we have learned; dialing a telephone number from memory is a test, so is cooking a meal, driving a car, tying shoes and even getting dressed. All of these day-to-day tasks are acquired knowledge and learned behaviors.

Preparation

The first step in test taking is to be well prepared. The previous section presented some ideas for successful studying and helping learners learn. Those steps for studying and learning are the means to being well prepared with the knowledge needed to pass a test successfully.

One way a group can facilitate learning is to have all individuals prepare a practice test on an assigned chapter. Each group member takes all tests, and then answers are checked. Group members find out where they need to focus more attention in their preparation for the real test.

Besides being prepared in the subject matter, there are other ways to prepare for a test. Be well rested; the mind functions much better when not fatigued. Make sure all the necessary materials are at hand before entering the classroom to avoid the frustration of searching for them.

Taking the Test

You are at your desk and the test is in front of you. The first thing to remember is to read each question carefully. By so doing some answers will suggest themselves during the reading process. The first question is not known, probably because of that test anxiety, but perhaps not. Go on to the next question and the next and so on until you find one question that you are absolutely sure you know. Continue through the test to the end, answering only the questions that you are positive you know. Often the first question you answer will unlock the brain freeze. Then go back and answer those questions you have to think about but know how to answer. Leave those questions you do not know for last. Often an answer to one of those tough ones can be found in another question.

With multiple choice questions, it is often possible to find the correct answer by eliminating the incorrect responses listed. True and false questions can be tricky. Beware of those that speak in absolutes such as "always" or "never." There are rarely any absolutes.

If you have studied thoroughly, and used your own anatomy to study, for example, using medical terms for your arms, legs, bones, and so on, you can use the "cheat sheet" that you carry around with you.

And, finally, remember this: a test is merely another tool in the learning process. Be prepared, be well rested and relax.

CHAPTER EXERCISES

CHAPTER 1   THE HUMAN BODY

CHAPTER OBJECTIVES

After studying this chapter, you should be able to:

1. Define the anatomic terms used to refer to the body in terms of directions and geometric planes.
2. Describe the major cavities of the body and the organs they contain.
3. Explain what a cell is.
4. Describe the major functions of the four types of human tissue.
5. List the major systems of the body, the organs they contain, and the functions of those systems.
6. Define the terms *anatomy* and *physiology*.
7. Define *homeostasis*.

ACTIVITIES

A. COMPLETION

Fill in the blank spaces with the correct term.

1. _____ is the structure of the body, and _____ is the function.

2. The four reference systems are _____, _____, _____ and _____ units.

3. The upper structures are considered to be _____, and a lower structure is _____.

4. An alternate term for anterior is _____.

5. An alternate term for dorsal is _____.

6. Toward the head is _____.

7. Nearest the origin is _____.

8. The opposite of the nearest point of attachment is _____.

9. The plane parallel to the median is the _____ plane.

10. Dividing the body into superior and inferior parts is the _____ plane.

11. Anterior and posterior portions are divided by the _____ plane.

12. Internal organs are the _____ of the body.

13. The dorsal cavity is divided into the _____ and the _____ cavities.

14. Between the pleural cavities is the _____.

15. The lining of the abdominal wall is the _____ _____.

16. _____ are the smallest units of life.

17. _____ is the liquid portion of a cell.

18. _____ is the study of diseases of the body.

19. The four categories of body tissue are _____, _____, _____ and _____.

20. _____ muscle is found only in the heart.

21. The integumentary system is made up of the _____ and the _____.

22. The balanced maintenance of the internal environment is _____.

23. The body is cooled by the action of _____ glands.

24. A group of organs performing a common function is called a _____.

25. Three kinds of muscle tissue are _____, _____ and _____.

B. MATCHING

Match the term on the right with the definition on the left.

26. _____ the belly side

27. _____ toward the head

28. _____ toward the tail

29. _____ frontal plane

30. _____ toward the side

31. _____ nearest the midline

32. _____ vertical division through the midline

33. _____ divide into superior and inferior

34. _____ second subdivision of the ventral cavity

35. _____ organ covering

36. _____ between the pleural cavities

37. _____ separates the abdominopelvic and thoracic cavities

38. _____ cavity surrounded by the rib cage

39. _____ solution containing groups of large molecules

40. _____ tissue covers surfaces

a. midsagittal

b. coronal

c. ventral

d. visceral

e. diaphragm

f. cranial

g. lateral

h. thoracic

i. caudal

j. epithelial

k. abdominopelvic

l. medial

m. colloidal

n. horizontal

o. mediastinum

C. KEY TERMS

Use the text to look up the following terms. Write the definition or explanation.

41. Abdominopelvic cavity: _____

_____

42. Cardiovascular system: _____

_____

43. Cephalad: _____

_____

44. Connective tissue: _____

_____

45. Coronal: _____

_____

46. Distal: _____

_____

47. Dorsal: _____

_____

48. Endocrine system: _____

_____

49. Inferior: _____

_____

50. Integumentary system: _____

_____

51. Lymphatic system: _____

_____

52. Mediastinum: _____

_____

53. Pericardial cavity: _____

_____

54. Pleural cavity: _____

_____

55. Protoplasm: _____

_____

56 Proximal: _____

_____

57. Reproductive system: _____

_____

58. Sagittal: _____

_____

59. Sebaceous glands: _____

_____

60. Spinal cavity: _____

_____

61. Thoracic cavity: _____

_____

62. Transverse: _____

_____

63. Urinary system: _____

_____

D. LABELING EXERCISE

64. Label the planes as indicated in Figure 1-1.

a. _____

b. _____

c. _____

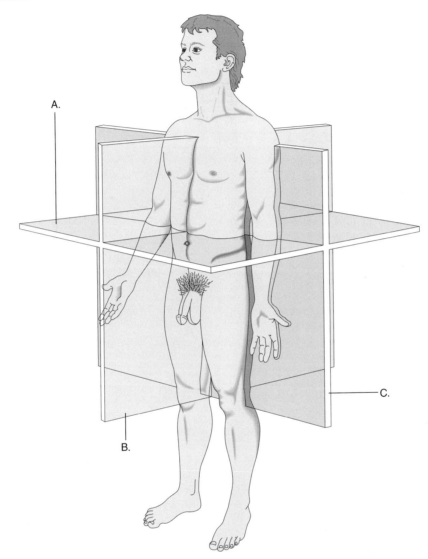

65. Label the directional terms as indicated in Figure 1-2.

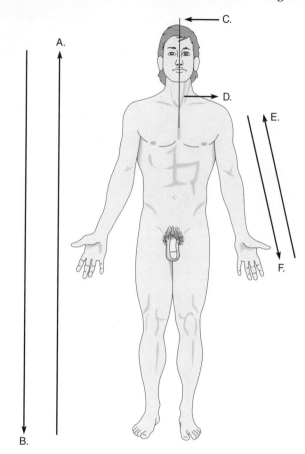

a. _____

b. _____

c. _____

d. _____

e. _____

f. _____

E. COLORING EXERCISE

66. Using Figure 1-3, color the dorsal cavities red, the abdominal cavity green, the pelvic cavity blue and the thoracic cavity yellow.

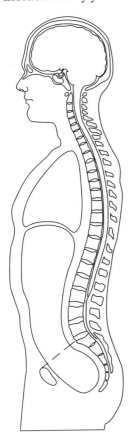

F. CRITICAL THINKING

Answer the following questions in complete sentences.

67. Why does the tongue have taste buds?

68. Why is it necessary to have reference positions of the body?

69. Why are the mammary glands on the anterior?

70. What do you think a bilateral tubalectomy means?

71. Which system is not needed for survival of the individual?

72. Explain the organization of the body.

73. Explain the "negative feedback loop" as it pertains to homeostasis.

74. Why does our heart pump faster when we run?

75. Which systems excrete waste?

76. Why do we have sebaceous glands?

G. CROSSWORD PUZZLE

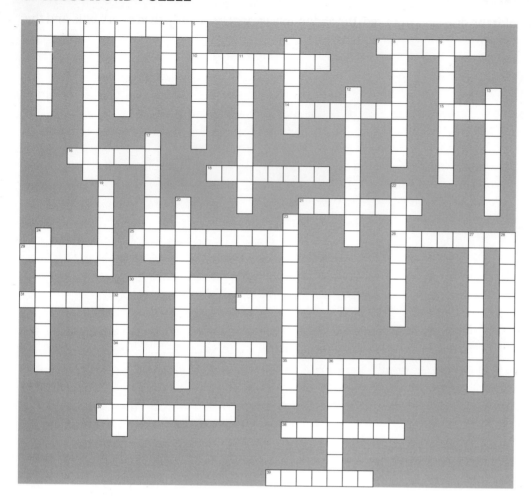

Complete the crossword puzzle using the following clues.

ACROSS

1. A healthy body
7. Internal organs
10. Toward the back
14. Toward the front
15. Basic unit
16. To the tail
18. Cavity wall
21. Cooling process
25. System that brings air to and from the lungs
26. Cavity containing the lungs
29. Produced by the salivary glands
30. Heart muscle

DOWN

1. William discovered circulation
2. Surface cover
3. Intestinal muscle
4. Senses temperature and pressure
5. Above
6. Farthest
8. Below
9. Ductless gland
11. Horizontal plane
12. Cell liquid
13. Glycogen to glucose
17. Animal starch
19. Back side

ACROSS

31. Divides the front and back

33. Goes with superior

34. Function of body parts

35. Body structure

37. Separates the chest and abdomen

38. Right and left parts

39. Blood glucose to the liver

DOWN

20. Not needed for body survival

22. Studies body structure

23. Temperature control

24. Diseases of the body

27. Tissue that binds and supports

28. Big molecule solution

32. Immune system

36. Nearest

CHAPTER QUIZ

1. The first person to correctly illustrate the human skeleton was
   a. William Harvey
   b. Andreas Vesalius
   c. Claude Bernard
   d. Jonas Salk
   e. Leonardo da Vinci

2. Salivary glands produce saliva, which contains
   a. carbohydrates
   b. HCl
   c. glucose
   d. enzymes
   e. pepsin

3. When referring to terms of direction, the human body is erect and facing
   a. posteriorly
   b. backward
   c. laterally
   d. horizontally
   e. forward

4. The study of diseases is called
   a. pathology
   b. physiology
   c. anatomy
   d. geology
   e. hematology

5. What position is the thoracic cavity in relation to the abdominal cavity?
   a. superior
   b. inferior
   c. lateral
   d. posterior
   e. ventral

6. Cranial is synonymous with
   a. lateral
   b. caudal
   c. superior
   d. inferior
   e. dorsal

7. The term that best describes the direction nearest to the midline of the body is
   a. superior
   b. sagittal
   c. medial
   d. inferior
   e. dorsal

8. With relation to the ankle, the knee is
   a. distal
   b. proximal
   c. lateral
   d. inferior
   e. caudal

9. With relation to the elbow, the wrist is
   a. distal
   b. proximal
   c. lateral
   d. superior
   e. caudal

10. Any plane parallel to the median plane is
    a. medial
    b. sagittal
    c. transverse
    d. dorsal
    e. ventral

11. A cut through the long axis of an organ is called what kind of section?
    a. distal
    b. transverse
    c. longitudinal
    d. horizontal
    e. coronal

12. A cut at right angles to the long axis is referred to as
    a. distal
    b. transverse
    c. horizontal
    d. longitudinal
    e. coronal

13. The body has how many major cavities?
    a. 2
    b. 4
    c. 6
    d. 8
    e. 10

14. The dorsal cavity contains organs of which system?
    a. muscular
    b. nervous
    c. endocrine
    d. respiratory
    e. digestive

15. The ventral cavity contains organs that are involved in maintaining
    a. feedback
    b. heartbeat
    c. homeostasis
    d. hormones
    e. growth

16. The heart in its sac resides in which cavity?
    a. dorsal
    b. coronal
    c. cranial
    d. pericardial
    e. abdominopelvic

17. The ovaries and uterus in women are contained in which cavity?
    a. dorsal
    b. thoracic
    c. abdominopelvic
    d. mediastinum
    e. pleural

18. The membrane lining the pleural wall is the
    a. parietal pleural
    b. visceral pleural
    c. parietal peritoneum
    d. visceral peritoneum
    e. parietal cranial

19. The membrane covering the abdominal organs is the
    a. parietal pleural
    b. visceral pleural
    c. parietal peritoneum
    d. visceral peritoneum
    e. parietal cranial

20. The membrane covering the lungs is the
    a. parietal pleural
    b. visceral pleural
    c. parietal peritoneum
    d. visceral peritoneum
    e. parietal cranial

21. The basic unit of biologic organization is the cell. Cells grouped together make up
    a. organs
    b. tissues
    c. systems
    d. protoplasm
    e. organelles

22. Mitochondria, ribosomes, and lyosomes are considered
    a. cells
    b. protoplasm
    c. organs
    d. tissue
    e. organelles

23. The type of tissue with little, if any, intercellular material is
    a. muscle
    b. nervous
    c. bone
    d. connective
    e. epithelial

24. The type of tissue having cells that produce elastin and collagen is
    a. muscle
    b. nervous
    c. hair
    d. connective
    e. epithelial

25. Which type of tissue has cells so long that they are called fibers?
    a. muscle
    b. nervous
    c. hair
    d. connective
    e. epithelial

26. Which system has organs functioning as levers?
    a. integumentary
    b. skeletal
    c. muscular
    d. nervous
    e. endocrine

27. Which system is composed of two layers?
    a. integumentary
    b. skeletal
    c. muscular
    d. nervous
    e. endocrine

28. Fibrous connective tissue is known as
    a. tendons
    b. cartilage
    c. dermis
    d. fasciae
    e. epidermis

29. Interpreting stimuli from the external environment is the function of which system?
    a. integumentary
    b. skeletal
    c. muscular
    d. nervous
    e. endocrine

30. Which of the following systems has as one of its functions the elimination of waste?
    a. lymphatic
    b. endocrine
    c. skeletal
    d. respiratory
    e. nervous

31. Of the following hormones, which one moves excess sugar into the liver?
    a. glycogen
    b. glucagon
    c. renin
    d. insulin
    e. thyroxin

32. Of the following, which is the best example of the negative feedback loop?
    a. eating
    b. swallowing
    c. walking
    d. sweating
    e. watching TV

33. Which of the following is NOT a function of the integumentary system?
    a. protection
    b. movement
    c. insulation
    d. water regulation
    e. temperature regulation

34. Which of the following is NOT a part of the lymphatic system?
    a. liver
    b. spleen
    c. lymph nodes
    d. tonsils
    e. thymus gland

35. Which cavity contains the brain and spinal cord?
    a. ventral
    b. dorsal
    c. pleural
    d. thoracic
    e. abdominopelvic

CHAPTER 2   THE CHEMISTRY OF LIFE

CHAPTER OBJECTIVES

After studying this chapter, you should be able to:

1. Define the structure of an atom and its component subatomic particles.
2. List the major chemical elements found in living systems.
3. Compare the differences between ionic and covalent bonding and how molecules formed by either ionic or covalent bonds react in water.
4. Understand the basic chemical structure of water, carbon dioxide and oxygen gas, ammonia, the mineral salts, carbohydrates, lipids, proteins, the nucleic acids DNA and RNA, and ATP and their role in living.
5. Explain the difference between diffusion, osmosis and active transport and their role in maintaining cellular structure and function.
6. Define *pH* and its significance in the human body.
7. Explain why water is so important to the body
8. Define the terms *acid*, *base* and *salt*.
9. Explain how the numbers in the pH scale relate to acidity and alkalinity.

ACTIVITIES

A. COMPLETION

Fill in the blank spaces with the correct term.

1. In the digestive process, complex foods are broken down into simpler substances like _____.

2. Sugar is eventually converted into a kind of chemical fuel called _____ _____.

3. All living and nonliving things are made of _____.

4. There are _____ natural elements.

5. _____ are the smallest particles of an element that keep all the characteristics of an element.

6. The nucleus of an atom contains a _____ and a _____.

7. The theory about matter and atoms was proposed by _____ _____.

8. Life on earth is based on the _____ atom.

9. Different kinds of atoms of the same element are called _____.

10. _____ has two electrons in the first level and six in the second.

11. When atoms combine chemically, they form _____.

12. A combination of two or more different elements is called a _____.

13. An _____ bond is formed when one atom gains electrons and another loses one.

14. _____ charged ions are attracted to _____ charged ions.

15. In _____ bonds, atoms share electrons.

16. A very weak bond is the _____ bond.

17. Molecules furnishing electrons are called _____.

18. Molecules gaining electrons are called _____.

19. Cells contain approximately _____ to _____ % water.

20. Digestion of food requires _____ to break down larger molecules.

21. _____ _____ contains one carbon atom and two oxygen atoms.

22. _____ comes from the decomposition of proteins.

23. The smallest carbohydrates are the _____ _____.

24. Two five-carbon sugars are _____ and _____.

25. Two six-carbon sugars are _____ and _____.

26. In the body, 95% of fats are _____.

27. Triglycerides are now called _____.

28. Triglycerides consist of _____ and _____ _____.

29. _____ increase the rate of a chemical reaction without being affected by it.

30. The three pyrimidine nitrogen bases are _____, _____ and _____.

31. ATP is made by putting together ADP with a _____ group.

32. The movement through a medium from high concentration to low concentration is called _____.

33. If the solution inside a cell and outside a cell are the same, it is _____.

34. The negative logarithm of the hydrogen ion concentration in a solution is _____.

35. A _____ is a substance that acts as a reservoir for hydrogen ions.

B. MATCHING

Match the term on the right with the definition on the left.

36. _____ CO_2 plus H_2O a. RNA

37. _____ combine with H+ ions in water   b. ions

38. _____ move materials against concentration   c. carbonic acids

39. _____ special kind of diffusion   d. DNA

40. _____ movement by random collision of molecules   e. unsaturated

41. _____ fuel for cell machinery   f. amino acids

42. _____ nucleic acid   g. base

43. _____ structurally related to DNA   h. osmosis

44. _____ build protein   i. glycogen

45. _____ fatty acid with one covalent bond   j. solvent

46. _____ carbon chain with more than one bond   k. atomic number

47. _____ substance insoluble in water   l. hydrolysis

48. _____ animal starch   m. diffusion

49. _____ composed of small ions   n. active transport

50. _____ medium for other reaction to occur in o. mineral salts

51. _____ H$_2$O helps to digest   p. ATP

52. _____ ability to do work   q. electron

53. _____ charged atom   r. lipid

54. _____ particles that orbit the atom nucleus s. saturated

55. _____ number of protons or electrons   t. energy

C. KEY TERMS

Use the text to look up the following terms. Write the definition or explanation.

56. Active transport: _____

_____

57. Amine group: _____

_____

58. Ammonia: _____

_____

59. Brownian movement: _____

_____

60. Carbohydrate: _____

_____

61. Carboxyl group: _____

_____

62. Compound: _____

_____

63. Covalent bond: _____

_____

64. Deoxyribonucleic acid: _____

_____

65. Electron carrier: _____

_____

66. Electron levels: _____

_____

67. Electrons: _____

_____

68. Fatty acid: _____

_____

69. Glycerol: _____

_____

70. Hydrogen bond: _____

_____

71. Hydroxyl group: _____

_____

72. Hypotonic group: _____

_____

73. Ion: _____

_____

74. Ionic bond: _____

_____

75. Mineral salts: _____

_____

76. Molecule: _____

_____

77. Neutron: _____

_____

78. Nucleotide: _____

_____

79. Orbitals: _____

_____

80. Primary structure: _____

_____

81. Purine: _____

_____

82. Selectively permeable membrane: _____

_____

83. Solute: _____

_____

84. Solvent: _____

_____

85. Unsaturated: _____

_____

D. LABELING EXERCISE

86. Label the structure as indicated in Figure 2-1.

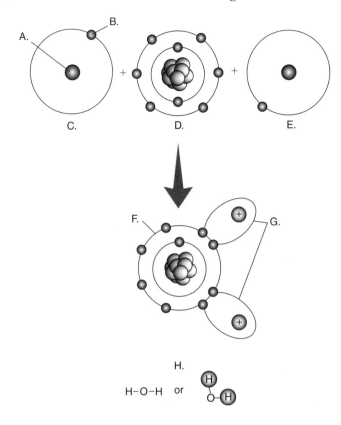

H–O–H   or

a. _____

b. _____

c. _____

d. _____

e. _____

f. _____

g. _____

h. _____

E. COLORING EXERCISE

There is no coloring exercise in this chapter.

F. CRITICAL THINKING

Answer the following questions in complete sentences.

87. Why do students of anatomy and physiology have to have a basic knowledge of chemistry?

88. Why are atoms never created or destroyed during a chemical reaction?

89. Why are water molecules polar?

90. Why do we not smell ice cream as well as we smell baking bread?

91. Differentiate the four types of protein structure.

92. Why is ATP necessary for cell nutrition?

93. How are chemical bonds formed?

94. Why is the amount of energy necessary to keep some atoms together so high?

95. Why do ionic bonded molecules disassociate in water?

96. Why do we need to exhale CO_2 quickly?

97. Why are animals dependent on plants for survival?

G. CROSSWORD PUZZLE

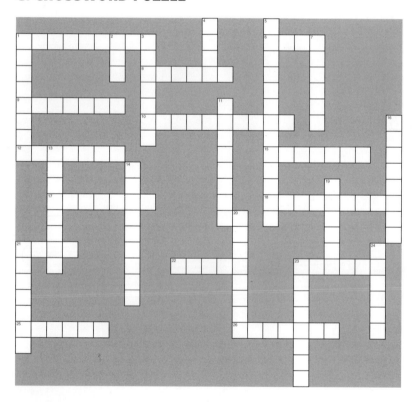

Complete the crossword puzzle using the following clues.

ACROSS

1. They orbit the nucleus

6. Smallest particles of elements

8. Insoluble in water

9. Protein catalysts

10. Basic structure of nucleic acid

12. Table sugar

15. Water through a membrane

DOWN

1. There are 92 naturals

2. Suffix denoting sugar

3. Medium for reaction to occur

4. Excess hydrogen ion in water

5. Cell respiration waste

7. All living and nonliving things are made of this

11. Bond where atoms share electrons

ACROSS

17. Adenine and guanine

18. Perfume through air

21. Charged atoms

22. Most abundant substance in cells

23. Found in all living matter

25. Positively charged particle

26. Has no charge

DOWN

13. Two or more elements

14. Molecular structure science

16. Normal saline solution

19. Reservoir for hydrogen ions

20. Essential element in amino acids

21. Same element, different atom

23. Needed for nerve transmission

24. The ability to do work

CHAPTER QUIZ

1. The use of water in the process of digestion is called
   a. hydrolysis
   b. osmosis
   c. chemical reaction
   d. photosynthesis
   e. diffusion

2. Primary substances from which all other things are constructed are called
   a. cells
   b. mineral salts
   c. compounds
   d. elements
   e. ATP

3. Atomic theory was a result of a proposal by
   a. Dimitri Mendeleev
   b. William Harvey
   c. Sir Robert Brown
   d. John Dalton
   e. Leonardo Da Vinci

4. Atoms of two or more elements form
   a. proteins
   b. amino acids
   c. protons
   d. compounds
   e. electrons

5. Chemistry that studies the nature of the carbon atom is
   a. organic
   b. physical
   c. atomic
   d. inorganic
   e. elemental

6. C12, C13 and C14 are considered
   a. ions
   b. molecules
   c. compounds
   d. isotonic
   e. isotopes

7. A radioactive isotope used to treat disorders of the thyroid gland is
   a. calcium
   b. chlorine
   c. sodium
   d. potassium
   e. iodine

8. A compound can also be a(n)
   a. electron
   b. molecule
   c. element
   d. proton
   e. atom

9. Sodium chloride is common
   a. sugar
   b. protein
   c. salt
   d. meat
   e. water

10. Which of the following is NOT a mineral salt?
    a. sodium
    b. potassium
    c. nitrogen
    d. calcium
    e. chloride

11. Weak bonds forming a bridge between water molecules are called
    a. ionic bonds
    b. hydrogen bonds
    c. covalent bonds
    d. molecule bonds
    e. atomic bonds

12. When two oxygen atoms are covalently bonded together, we have
    a. water
    b. carboxyl
    c. molecular oxygen
    d. carbon dioxide
    e. hydroxyl group

13. An important element in ammonia is
    a. potassium
    b. sulphur
    c. phosphate
    d. nitrogen
    e. ATP

14. What percentage of our atmosphere is oxygen?
    a. 14%
    b. 60%
    c. 100%
    d. 30%
    e. 21%

15. Which of the following mineral salts is necessary to produce ATP?
    a. sodium
    b. potassium
    c. calcium
    d. chloride
    e. phosphate

16. Which of the following is a disaccharide?
    a. glycogen
    b. glucose
    c. ribose
    d. sucrose
    e. fructose

17. Which of the following is NOT a lipid?
    a. glucose
    b. fats
    c. phospholipid
    d. steroids
    e. prostaglandin

18. Bonds formed between different amino acids to make protein are
    a. ionic
    b. hydrogen
    c. peptide
    d. carboxyl
    e. lipid

19. Chemical reactions would not occur in cells without
    a. enzymes
    b. lipids
    c. amines
    d. sodium
    e. acid

20. RNA molecules are a single chain of
    a. mineral
    b. nucleotides
    c. glycerol
    d. amines
    e. purines

21. Which of the following is NOT a part of a DNA molecule?
    a. adenine
    b. cytosine
    c. uracil
    d. thymine
    e. guanine

22. The energy of the ATP molecule is stored in which phosphate group?
    a. first/second
    b. second/third
    c. third/fourth
    d. fourth/fifth
    e. fifth/sixth

23. Which of the following is NOT a method of passing materials through a cell membrane?
    a. diffusion
    b. hydrolysis
    c. active transport
    d. osmosis
    e. none of the above

24. Random collision of diffusing molecules is known as the
    a. haversian canal
    b. down flow
    c. brownian movement
    d. Hook's movement
    e. Monk's movement

25. A normal saline solution is
    a. hypertonic
    b. isotonic
    c. sweet
    d. ionic
    e. hypotonic

26. Pure water has a pH of
    a. 8
    b. 10
    c. 0.08
    d. 7
    e. 6

27. A substance that combines with H⁺ ions in water is
    a. buffer
    b. base
    c. acid
    d. alkaloid
    e. hydroxyl

28. A substance that combines with H⁺ ions in water is a(n)
    a. buffer
    b. base
    c. acid
    d. alkaloid
    e. hydroxyl

29. Which is more acidic?
    a. blood
    b. urine
    c. gastric juice
    d. tomato juice
    e. milk

30. How many amino acids are there?
    a. 10
    b. 20
    c. 30
    d. 40
    e. 50

CHAPTER 3   CELL STRUCTURE

CHAPTER OBJECTIVES

After studying this chapter, you should be able to:

1. Name the major contributors to the cell theory.
2. Explain the molecular structure of a cell membrane.
3. Describe the structure and function of cellular organelles.
4. Explain the significance and process of protein synthesis.

ACTIVITIES

A. COMPLETION

Fill in the blank spaces with the correct term.

1. Higher cells like those of the body are called _____.

2. Cells without organelles are called _____.

3. The sperm cell has a _____ to propel it.

4. Cells are measured in terms of _____.

5. Living cells were first observed by a man named _____.

6. The cell membrane is called the _____.

7. Protoplasm inside the nucleus is called _____.

8. A molecule with unequal distribution of bonding electrons is said to be _____.

9. Compounds that do not readily dissolve in water are _____.

10. Human body cells contain _____ chromosomes.

11. A spherical particle within the nucleoplasm is the _____.

12. The folds of the inner membrane of the mitochondria are called _____.

13. All cells have approximately the same number of _____.

14. In a cell, proteins are assembled from _____.

15. The expulsion of lysosome enzymes into cell cytoplasm is known as _____.

16. Membrane forming a collection of cavities is the _____ _____.

17. Rough ER is a site of _____ _____.

18. Point of collection for compounds to be secreted are _____ _____.

19. Messenger RNA attaches to _____ during protein synthesis.

20. It copies codes from the DNA molecule in the nucleus; it is called _____ RNA.

21. _____ RNA will go into the cytoplasm and collect amino acids.

22. Two centrioles are referred to as a _____.

23. Cellular organelles located on the surface are _____ and _____.

24. Euglena are propelled by a _____.

25. Paramecium is propelled by _____.

26. _____ cause plants to look green.

27. _____ occurs inside chloroplasts.

28. Layers of proteins, enzymes and chlorophyll make up the _____.

29. Plant cell walls are composed of _____.

30. Carotenoid pigments are _____ and _____.

B. MATCHING

Match the term on the right with the definition on the left.

31. _____ structure within protoplasm

32. _____ organelles for photosynthesis

33. _____ protoplasm inside nucleus

34. _____ one thousandth a millimeter

35. _____ attracts water

36. _____ repels water

37. _____ protoplasm outside nucleus

38. _____ dark threads in nucleus

39. _____ controls all cell functions

40. _____ contain digestive enzymes

41. _____ smooth ER

42. _____ resembles a stack of saucers

43. _____ foreign proteins

44. _____ protein make long hollow cylinders

45. _____ plants look green

a. chromatin

b. lysosome

c. organelles

d. Golgi body

e. antigens

f. chloroplasts

g. chlorophyll

h. micrometer

i. hydrophilic

j. cytoplasm

k. nucleoplasm

l. tubulin

m. hydrophobic

n. agranular

o. DNA

C. KEY TERMS

Use the text to look up the following terms. Write the definition or explanation.

46. Apoptosis: _____

_____

47. Carotene: _____

_____

48. Chromoplast: _____

_____

49. Cisternae: _____

_____

50. Deoxyribonucleic acid: _____

_____

51. Golgi apparatus: _____

_____

52. Leucoplasts: _____

_____

53. Messenger RNA: _____

_____

54. Microtubular: _____

_____

55. Nonpolar: _____

_____

56. Nucleolus: _____

_____

57. Plasma membrane: _____

_____

58. Polar: _____

_____

59. Prokaryotic: _____

_____

60. Protein synthesis: _____

_____

61. Ribonucleic acid: _____

_____

62. Transcription: _____

_____

63. Translation: _____

_____

64. Vacuoles: _____

_____

65. Xanthophyll: _____

_____

D. LABELING EXERCISE

66. Label the parts of the cell indicated in Figure 3-1.

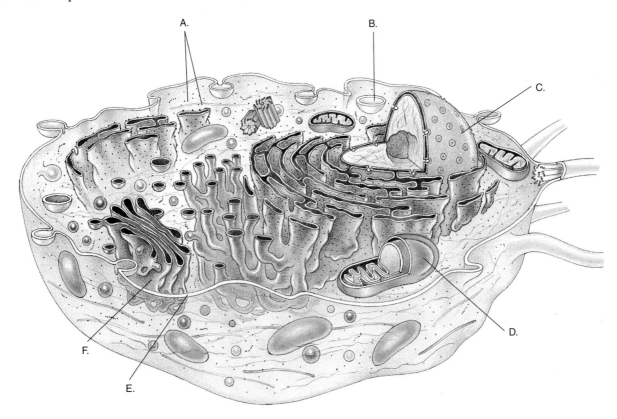

a. _____

b. _____

c. _____

d. _____

e. _____

f. _____

67. Label the chromosomal organization as indicated in Figure 3-2.

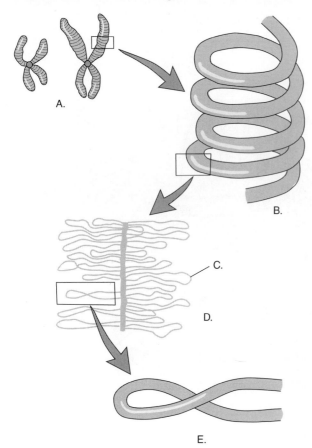

A.

B.

C.

D.

E.

a. _____

b. _____

c. _____

d. _____

e. _____

E. COLORING EXERCISE

68. Using Figure 3-3, color the chloroplasts green, the cell wall brown, the mitochondria blue and the cytoplasm gray.

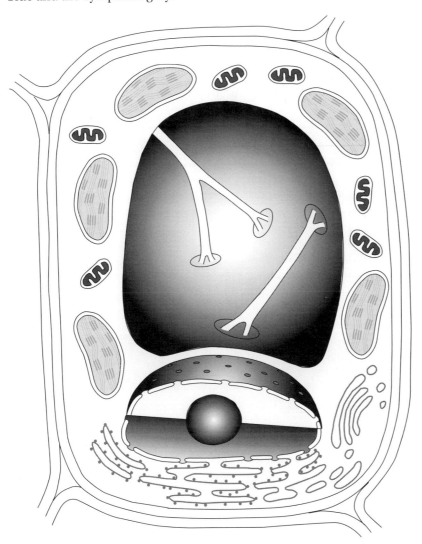

F. CRITICAL THINKING

Answer the following questions in complete sentences.

69. Explain the symbiotic relationship between plants and animals.

70. The invention of the microscope was necessary for the development of cell theory. What invention or process was needed before the microscope?

71. Why is water a major constituent of the body and how is it used?

72. Explain the relationship of DNA and RNA.

73. Normal cells contain 46 chromosomes. Which cells contain fewer, how many and why?

74. Why do muscle cells have mitochondria with cristae?

75. When is agranular ER attached to granular ER?

76. Why do plant cells have a cell wall made of cellulose?

G. CROSSWORD PUZZLE

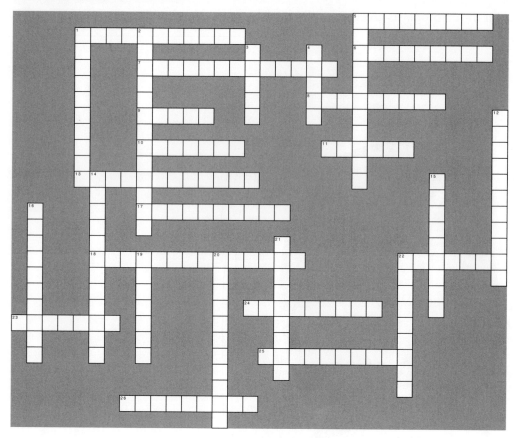

Complete the crossword puzzle using the following clues.

ACROSS

1. Cell membrane
5. Spherical with no membrane
6. Makes plant cell wall
7. Copying DNA code
8. Cell suicide
9. First described cells
10. Control center of cell
11. Stack of thylakoid
13. Plant cell plastid
17. Structures in cell protoplasm
18. Light energy to chemical energy
22. Inner folds of mitochondrion
23. Storage area in cell
24. Contain digestion enzymes
25. No pigment plastid
26. Flat saclike cisternae

DOWN

1. Like bacteria cells
2. Cell's powerhouse
3. Organelle like hair
4. Unequal bonding electrons
5. Protoplasm in nucleus
12. DNA and protein
14. Attracts water
15. Used in cell division
16. Colloidal cell liquid
19. Long hollow cylinders of protein
20. Matching of DNA codes
21. Responsible for protein synthesis
22. Cell's genetic material

CHAPTER QUIZ

1. Bacteria cells are
   a. organelles
   b. eukaryotic
   c. round
   d. prokaryotic
   e. none of the above

2. The most prominent structure in the cell is the
   a. mitochondrion
   b. nucleus
   c. ribosome
   d. lysosome
   e. vacuole

3. The first person to observe a living cell was
   a. Hooke
   b. Schwann
   c. Schleidon
   d. Harvey
   e. Leeuwenhoek

4. ATP is needed in cells for which process?
   a. diffusion
   b. active transport
   c. osmosis
   d. passage of water molecules
   e. passage of ions

5. Which of the following is NOT a function of protein in the cell membrane?
   a. ATP synthesis
   b. pass molecules and ions
   c. receptors for hormones
   d. identity markers
   e. sodium-potassium pump

6. Protoplasm is
   a. an organelle
   b. part of the cell membrane
   c. in the nucleus
   d. liquid portion of cell
   e. a hormone

7. Clumps of atoms distributed throughout a medium is a
   a. cytoplasm
   b. molecule
   c. solution
   d. nucleic acid
   e. colloid

8. A polar molecule has which of the following?
   a. O positive and H negative
   b. O and H no charge
   c. O neutral and H positive
   d. O negative and H positive
   e. H neutral and O positive

9. Compounds of unequal distribution of bonding electrons are said to be
   a. colloid
   b. soluble
   c. nonpolar
   d. clumping
   e. enzymes

10. Which of the following would NOT go into a solution?
    a. sodium
    b. potassium
    c. chlorine
    d. phosphorus
    e. none of the above

11. Which of the following are NOT colloidally suspended in the cytoplasm?
    a. proteins
    b. carbohydrates
    c. fats
    d. nucleic acid
    e. none of the above

12. Which of the following are NOT surrounded by a membrane?
    a. nucleus
    b. nucleolus
    c. animal cell
    d. vacuole
    e. plant cell

13. The code to make protein is found on the
    a. RNA
    b. ribosome
    c. mitochondria
    d. DNA
    e. lysosome

14. The genetic material of the cell is found in the
    a. chromatin
    b. RNA
    c. ribosomes
    d. nuclear membrane
    e. cisternae

15. There are many folds in the
    a. plasma membrane
    b. nuclear membrane
    c. mitochondrion membrane
    d. vacuole membrane
    e. plant membrane

16. Cellular respiration occurs on the
    a. RNA
    b. plasma membrane
    c. cristae
    d. cisternae
    e. lysosome

17. Mitochondria with many cristae will be found in which cells?
    a. skin
    b. blood
    c. lymph
    d. nerve
    e. muscle

18. Maintenance and repair of cellular components is a function of the
    a. lysosome
    b. mitochondria
    c. nucleolus
    d. ribosomes
    e. parallelism

19. Saclike or channel-like cisternae are found in the
    a. endoplasmic reticulum
    b. nucleus
    c. ribosomes
    d. mitochondria
    e. Golgi body

20. The site of protein synthesis in the cell is the
    a. Golgi body
    b. nucleus
    c. ribosome
    d. mitochondria
    e. endoplasmic reticulum

21. The concentration of compounds to be secreted is a function of the
    a. Golgi body
    b. nucleus
    c. ribosome
    d. mitochondria
    e. endoplasmic reticulum

22. The substance that gives plants a green color is
    a. carotene
    b. glucose
    c. chlorophyll
    d. xanthophyll
    e. cellulose

23. The substance that gives plants a red-orange color is
    a. carotene
    b. glucose
    c. chlorophyll
    d. xanthophyll
    e. cellulose

24. The fiber in our diet from plants is the substance
    a. carotene
    b. glucose
    c. chlorophyll
    d. xanthophyll
    e. cellulose

25. Protein synthesis relies on which of the following?
    a. grana
    b. leucoplasts
    c. mRNA
    d. vacuoles
    e. lamella

26. During protein synthesis amino acids are collected. The code for a particular amino acid is made possible by three bases using the element
    a. potassium
    b. nitrogen
    c. chlorine
    d. sulfur
    e. phosphorous

27. Centrioles function during
    a. protein synthesis
    b. digestion
    c. photosynthesis
    d. cell division
    e. ATP production

28. The number of plastids found in plant cells is
    a. 1
    b. 2
    c. 3
    d. 4
    e. 5

29. The process of photosynthesis occurs in the
    a. leucoplast
    b. nucleus
    c. xanthophyll
    d. chloroplast
    e. chromoplast

30. The nuclear membrane allows certain materials to leave the nucleus through
    a. pores
    b. tubules
    c. microtubules
    d. vacuoles
    e. cisternae

CHAPTER 4   CELLULAR METABOLISM AND REPRODUCTION: MITOSIS AND MEIOSIS

CHAPTER OBJECTIVES

After studying this chapter, you should be able to:

1. Define *metabolism*.
2. Describe the basic steps in glycolysis and indicate the major products and ATP production.
3. Describe the Krebs' citric acid cycle and its major products and ATP production.
4. Describe the electron transport system and how ATP is produced.
5. Compare glycolysis with anaerobic production of ATP in muscle cells and fermentation.
6. Explain how other food compounds besides glucose are used as energy sources.
7. Name the discoverers of the anatomy of the DNA molecule.
8. Know the basic structure of the DNA molecule.
9. Name the nitrogen base pairs and how they pair up in the DNA molecule.
10. Define the stages of the cell cycle.
11. Explain the significance of mitosis in the survival of the cell and growth in the human body.
12. Understand the significance of meiosis as a reduction of the genetic material and for the formation of the sex cells.

ACTIVITIES

A. COMPLETION

Fill in the blank spaces with the correct term.

1. To maintain structure and function, _____ _____ must occur in cells.

2. Total chemical changes occurring inside a cell is called _____.

3. _____ builds and requires energy.

4. _____ breaks down and releases energy.

5. These processes are called _____ _____.

6. The process using CO_2, H_2O, light and chlorophyll to produce food is called _____.

7. Anaerobic glucose decomposition in yeast is called _____.

8. _____ is the process for adding a phosphate to glucose during glycolysis.

9. _____ is the result of cleaving fructose diphosphate.

10. Glycolytic breakdown of one glucose molecule provides two _____ _____ molecules.

11. The transition from C_3 pyruvic acid to C_2 acetyl-CoA has a first transitional conversion of _____ _____.

12. The Krebs' citric acid cycle produces five acids in transition; they are _____, _____, _____, _____ and _____.

13. When yeast breaks down glucose, the resultant products are _____ _____, _____ _____ and _____.

14. During fermentation, the enzyme decarboxylase breaks down_____ _____ and _____.

15. Anaerobic breakdown of glucose in muscle cells produces _____ _____.

16. Fatty acids and glycerol are products of _____ digestion.

17. Digestion breaks down protein into _____ _____.

18. Meiosis occurs only in the _____.

19. Levine discovered that DNA contained _____ _____, _____ _____ _____, _____ and _____.

20. Two purines in DNA are _____ and _____.

21. Two pyrimidines in DNA are _____ and _____.

22. The four letters in the alphabet of life are _____, _____, _____ and _____.

23. The cell cycle's three stages are _____, _____ and _____.

24. Strands of DNA duplicate themselves during the _____ _____.

25. The four stages of mitosis are _____, _____, _____ and _____.

26. A _____ cell is an exact duplicate of a parent cell resulting from mitosis.

27. _____ _____ are a group of microtubules between cell poles.

28. Chromosomes first form a ring during _____.

29. The shortest and most dynamic phase is _____.

30. Actual cell division into two daughter cells is accomplished by a _____ _____.

31. During _____, a nuclear membrane forms around each group of daughter chromosomes.

32. The male gamete is the _____ and the female gamete is the _____.

33. Mitosis has one cell division; meiosis has _____.

34. There are _____ daughter cells produced during meiosis and each contains _____ chromosomes.

35. Meiosis resembles mitosis during its second stage; however, there is no duplication of _____.

B. MATCHING

Match the term on the right with the definition on the left.

36. _____ sex cells

37. _____ citric acid cycle

38. _____ defective cells spread

39. _____ two chromatids, one centromere

40. _____ cells divide continuously

41. _____ disruption of DNA code copying

42. _____ occurs in testes

43. _____ occurs in ovaries

44. _____ result in 4 haploid daughter cells

45. _____ chromosomes exchange genetic material

46. _____ full number of chromosomes

47. _____ forms new cell wall

48. _____ phase for cell division preparation

49. _____ always pairs with thymine

50. _____ always pairs with cytosine

51. _____ DNA a winding staircase

52. _____ 2 ATP produced

53. _____ 6 ATP produced

54. _____ energy from glucose

55. _____ nicotinamide adenine dinucleotide

a. crossing over

b. G_2

c. spermatogenesis

d. diploid

e. gametes

f. telophase II

g. adenine

h. Rosalind Franklin

i. Krebs'

j. metaphase II

k. mutation

l. oogenesis

m. NAD

n. cancer

o. ATP

p. $2NADH_2$

q. metastasize

r. cell plate

s. guanine

t. glycolysis

C. KEY TERMS

Use the text to look up the following terms. Write the definition or explanation.

56. Aerobic: _____

_____

57. Alpha-ketoglutaric acid: _____

_____

58. Anaerobic respiration: _____

_____

59. Cellular respiration metabolism: _____

_____

60. Chiasmata: _____

_____

61. Chromatid: _____

_____

62. Chromatin: _____

_____

63. Cleavage furrow: _____

_____

64. Crossing over: _____

_____

65. Electron transfer/transport system: _____

_____

66. Fermentation: _____

_____

67. Flavin adenine dinucleotide: _____

_____

68. Gametogenesis: _____

_____

69. Glycolysis: _____

_____

70. Haploid: _____

_____

71. Kinetochore: _____

_____

72. Lactic acid: _____

_____

73. Metastasize: _____

_____

74. Mutation: _____

_____

75. Phosphoglyceraldehyde (PGAL): _____

_____

76. Phosphorylation: _____

_____

77. Polar bodies: _____

_____

78. Quinone: _____

_____

79. Synapsis: _____

_____

80. Tetrad: _____

_____

D. LABELING EXERCISE

81. Label the cellular respiration steps as indicated in Figure 4-1.

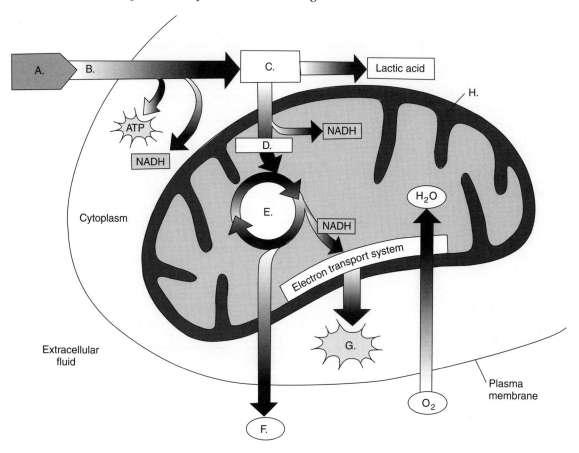

a. _____

b. _____

c. _____

d. _____

e. _____

f. _____

g. _____

h. _____

82. Label the mitosis phase as indicated in Figure 4-2.

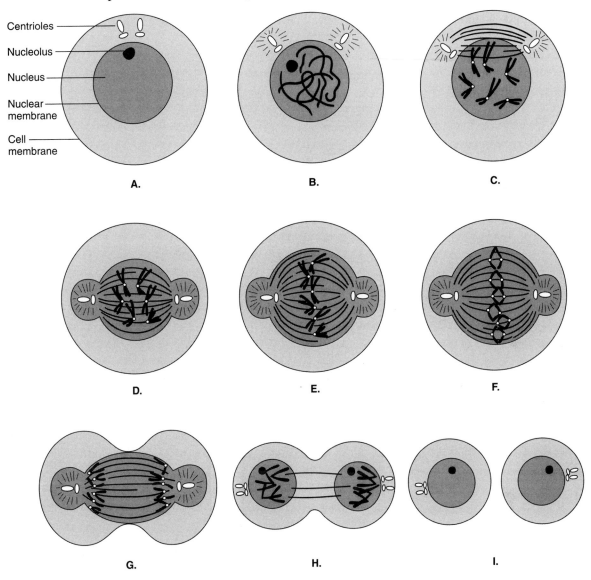

a. _____
b. _____
c. _____
d. _____
e. _____
f. _____
g. _____
h. _____
i. _____

E. COLORING EXERCISE

83. Using Figure 4-3, color the thymine molecule yellow, the adenine blue, the guanine green and the cytosine orange.

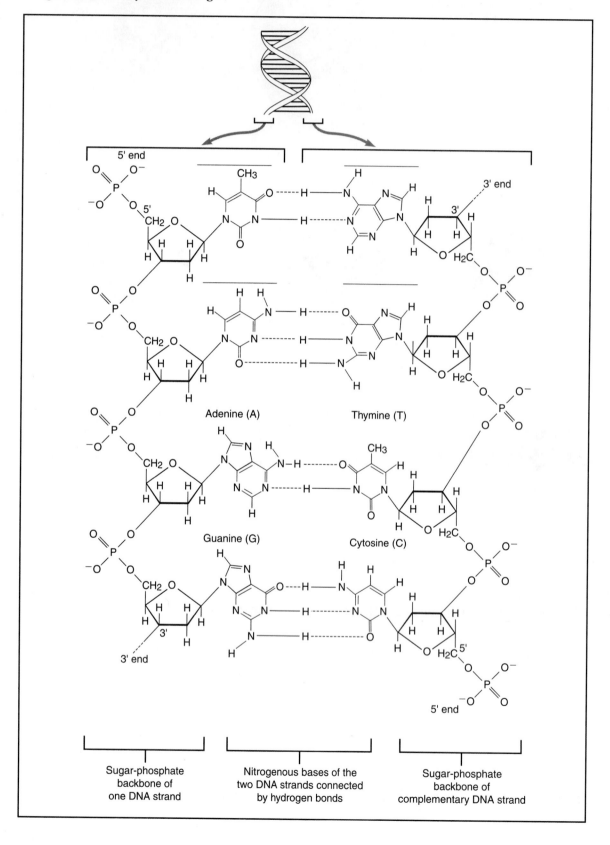

Adenine (A)   Thymine (T)

Guanine (G)   Cytosine (C)

Sugar-phosphate backbone of one DNA strand

Nitrogenous bases of the two DNA strands connected by hydrogen bonds

Sugar-phosphate backbone of complementary DNA strand

84. Using Figure 4-4, color the deoxyribose red. Connect the TA, AT, GC and CG with their respective colors (those used in Figure 4-3).

S = Deoxyribose, P = Phosphate, C = Cytosine,
G = Guanine, A = Adenine, T = Thymine

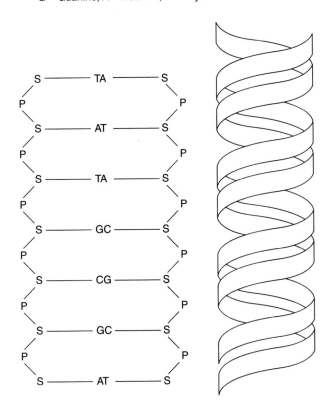

F. CRITICAL THINKING

Answer the following questions in complete sentences.

85. Why do we continue to breathe hard after exercise?

86. Why is meiosis necessary?

87. Explain the difference between anabolism and catabolism.

88. Explain the plant/animal energy cycle.

89. Why is the biochemical production of energy more efficient than that of a man-made machine?

90. Why do alanine and lactic acid enter the cellular furnace at the pyruvic acid stage?

91. Why was the revelation of Rosalind Franklin, James Watson and Francis Crick so important?

92. What is a gene?

93. Why is the genome project so important?

94. Is interphase really a resting phase? Explain.

95. Which of the three cellular reproduction careers interest you the most? Why?

G. CROSSWORD PUZZLE

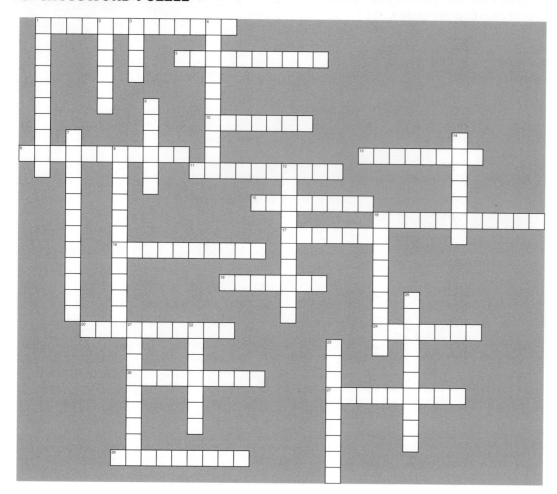

Complete the crossword puzzle using the following clues.

ACROSS
1. Formation of sex cells
5. Cellular respiration
6. Disk of protein
10. 23 chromosomes
11. Pinched in area
13. Friedreich the chemist
15. Disruption of genetic code
16. Phosphate group
17. Bone cancer
18. Organelle duplication
19. Reduction division
20. Cancer causing
24. Normal cell division

DOWN
1. Cell respiration
2. Visible pair of chromosomes
3. Sequence of organic nitrogen
4. Between phases
7. Yeast cells feed on glucose
8. Exchange genetic material
9. Fertilized egg
12. Tumor moves
14. Needing oxygen
18. From epithelial tissue
21. Dark threads
22. Pairs with cytosine
23. X-shaped structure

ACROSS

26. Formation of female egg

27. Builds molecules

28. Without oxygen

DOWN

25. Break down molecule

CHAPTER QUIZ

1. The complete chemical process of chemical change in a cell is called
   a. anabolism
   b. metabolism
   c. catabolism
   d. glycolysis
   e. digestion

2. Breaking down molecules with a release of energy is
   a. anabolism
   b. metabolism
   c. catabolism
   d. glycolysis
   e. digestion

3. Using energy to construct molecular material is
   a. anabolism
   b. metabolism
   c. catabolism
   d. glycolysis
   e. digestion

4. The ultimate source of food is the result of a process called
   a. metabolism
   b. glycolysis
   c. photosynthesis
   d. aerobics
   e. mitosis

5. Which of the following is NOT used in photosynthesis?
   a. H_2O
   b. $6CO_2$
   c. light
   d. chlorophyll
   e. O_2

6. The first step in the process of breaking down a glucose molecule is
   a. digestion
   b. aerobic
   c. anabolism
   d. glycolysis
   e. photosynthesis

7. During the latter part of prolonged exercise, human muscles start to break down glucose by the process of
   a. anaerobic respiration
   b. aerobic respiration
   c. respiration
   d. anabolism
   e. electron transport

8. During glycolysis, glucose is broken down to
   a. lactic acid
   b. malic acid
   c. pyruvic acid
   d. citric acid
   e. folic acid

9. Phosphoglyceride is formed in which step of glycolysis?
   a. first
   b. second
   c. third
   d. fourth
   e. fifth

10. When the phosphoglyceric acids are broken down, how many ATP molecules are formed?
    a. 2
    b. 4
    c. 6
    d. 8
    e. 10

11. Aerobic glycolysis produces how many molecules of ATP?
    a. 2
    b. 4
    c. 6
    d. 8
    e. 10

12. During the first part of Krebs' citric acid cycle, pyruvic acid is converted to
    a. acetic acid
    b. lactic acid
    c. oxaloacetic acid
    d. malic acid
    e. succinic acid

13. The Krebs' citric acid cycle takes place in the
    a. lysosome
    b. vacuoles
    c. nucleus
    d. mitochondria
    e. ribosomes

14. Alpha-ketoglutaric acid is broken down into
    a. malic acid
    b. pyruvic acid
    c. acetic acid
    d. succinic acid
    e. folic acid

15. The electrons of which element are the primary substance carried by the electron transport system?
    a. hydrogen
    b. oxygen
    c. phosphorus
    d. sulfur
    e. potassium

16. The final product of fermentation is
    a. malic acid
    b. alcohol
    c. yeast
    d. sugar
    e. bread

17. During anaerobic production of ATP in muscle, which acid is formed?
    a. pyruvic
    b. folic
    c. malic
    d. oxaloacetic
    e. lactic

18. Which of the following is NOT a carbohydrate?
    a. glucose
    b. starch
    c. glycogen
    d. monosaccharides
    e. glycerol

19. Duplication of cellular organelles is called
    a. cytokinesis
    b. mitosis
    c. meiosis
    d. phosphorylation

20. The two purines are composed of
    a. folic acid and oxygen
    b. thymine and cytosine
    c. adenine and guanine
    d. cytosine and adenine
    e. adenine and thymine

21. The two pyrimidines are composed of
    a. folic acid and oxygen
    b. thymine and cytosine
    c. adenine and guanine
    d. cytosine and adenine
    e. adenine and thymine

22. Certain cells divide only if damaged; they are
    a. skin cells
    b. hair cells
    c. liver cells
    d. blood cells
    e. muscle cells

23. The longest phase of the cell cycle is
    a. prophase
    b. telophase
    c. cytokinesis
    d. interphase
    e. mitosis

24. Which of the following is NOT a stage of mitosis?
    a. interphase
    b. prophase
    c. metaphase
    d. anaphase
    e. telophase

25. Which of the following is NOT part of prophase?
    a. aster
    b. kinetochore
    c. centromere
    d. spindle fiber
    e. none of the above

26. All of the following are a part of metaphase EXCEPT
    a. aster
    b. kinetochore
    c. centromere
    d. spindle fiber
    e. none of the above

27. Which of the following is the shortest phase of mitosis?
    a. interphase
    b. prophase
    c. metaphase
    d. anaphase
    e. telophase

28. The final stage of mitosis is
    a. interphase
    b. telophase
    c. prophase
    d. anaphase
    e. metaphase

29. A cell with 23 chromosomes is
    a. diploid
    b. muscle
    c. zygote
    d. haploid
    e. gonad

30. Which of the following cancers is considered hereditary?
    a. colon
    b. lung
    c. skin
    d. breast
    e. none of the above

CHAPTER 5 TISSUES

CHAPTER OBJECTIVES

After studying this chapter, you should be able to:

1. Classify epithelial tissue based on shape and arrangement and give examples.
2. Name the types of glands in the body and give examples.
3. Name the functions of connective tissue.
4. Compare epithelial tissue with connective tissue in terms of cell arrangement and interstitial materials.
5. Name the three major types of connective tissue and give examples.
6. List the functions of epithelial tissue.
7. List the three types of muscle and describe each based on structure and function.
8. Describe the anatomy of a neuron and the function of nervous tissue.

ACTIVITIES

A. COMPLETION

Fill in the blank spaces with the correct term.

1. One who specializes in analyzing tissue samples looking for clues that help solve crimes is a/an _____ _____.

2. Groups of cells with similar function form _____.

3. The four types of tissue in the human body are _____, _____, _____ and _____.

4. The four functions of epithelial tissue are _____, _____, _____ and _____.

5. Tall and rectangular cells are called _____.

6. A simple arrangement of epithelial cells can be found in the _____, _____ and _____.

7. The epithelial cell arrangement found lining the throat is called _____.

8. Mucous membranes are usually _____.

9. Glandular tissue forms _____ and _____ glands.

10. The tissue lining the circulatory system is _____.

11. The mesothelium is also called _____ tissue.

12. The type of tissue providing for movement and support is _____.

13. This type of tissue has intercellular material called a _____.

14. Connective tissue has the subgroups called _____, _____ and _____.

15. The most widely distributed connective tissue is _____.

16. Areolar tissue has three main types of cells, _____, _____ and _____.

17. _____ tissue is fat.

18. Dense connective tissues bearing a regular arrangement of fibers are _____.

19. The connective tissue attaching bones to bones is called _____.

20. The tissue covering a muscle is _____.

21. Cells of cartilage are called _____.

22. Cartilage that has a matrix with no fibers is called _____.

23. Elastin fibers embedded in the matrix of this connective tissue give it the name _____ cartilage.

24. The dense connective tissue making up the teeth is named _____.

25. _____ is liquid tissue.

26. Mucus-secreting tissues are made up of _____ cells.

27. Marrow and lymphoid organs are referred to as _____ tissue.

28. Phagocytes are found in _____ tissue.

29. Three types of muscle tissue are _____, _____ and _____.

30. A neuron consists of an _____, a _____ _____ and a _____.

B. MATCHING

Match the term on the right with the definition of the left.

31. _____ study of tissue
32. _____ cells flat and irregular
33. _____ small cubes
34. _____ secrete mucus
35. _____ lines thoracic cavity
36. _____ lines abdominal cavity
37. _____ motile phagocytes
38. _____ anticoagulant
39. _____ wide flat tendon
40. _____ cartilage cavities
41. _____ cells lining liver
42. _____ phagocytic cell in nervous system
43. _____ ability to shorten and thicken
44. _____ pushes food along digestive tract
45. _____ striated muscle
46. _____ cells shorter than smooth
47. _____ ductless glands

a. heparin
b. Kupffer's
c. cardiac
d. histology
e. muscle tissue
f. lacunae
g. squamous
h. fibroblasts
i. cuboidal
j. pleura
k. endocrine
l. neurons
m. peritoneum
n. goblet cells
o. fibrocartilage
p. aponeurosis
q. neuroglia

48. _____ make fibers for repair   r. skeletal

49. _____ intervertebral disks   s. macrophages

50. _____ conducting cells   t. peristalsis

C. KEY TERMS

Use the text to look up the following terms. Write the definition or explanation.

51. Adipose: _____

_____

52. Axon: _____

_____

53. Basement membrane: _____

_____

54. Chondrocyte: _____

_____

55. Collagen: _____

_____

56. Compound exocrine glands: _____

_____

57. Connective tissue: _____

_____

58. Dendrite: _____

_____

59. Elastin: _____

_____

60. Endocardium: _____

_____

61. Exocrine glands: _____

_____

62. Histamine: _____

_____

63. Intercalated disks: _____

_____

64. Microglia: _____

_____

65. Parietal: _____

_____

66. Peristalsis: _____

_____

67. Phagocytic: _____

_____

68. Pseudostratified epithelial: _____

_____

69. Reticuloendothelial system: _____

_____

70. Serous tissue: _____

_____

71. Simple epithelial: _____

_____

72. Stratified epithelial: _____

_____

73. Synovial membrane: _____

_____

74. Transitional epithelial: _____

_____

75. Visceral: _____

_____

D. LABELING EXERCISE

76. Label Figure 5-1 as indicated.

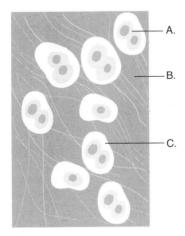

    a. _____

    b. _____

    c. _____

77. Label Figure 5-2 as indicated.

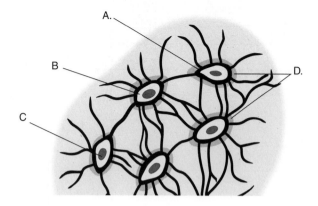

a. _____
b. _____
c. _____
d. _____

78. Label Figure 5-3 as indicated.

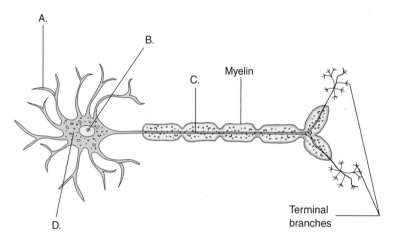

a. _____
b. _____
c. _____
d. _____

E. COLORING EXERCISE

79. Using Figure 5-4, color the erythrocytes red, thrombocytes green, lymphocyte blue, neutrophil yellow, monocyte brown, basophil orange and eosinophil pink.

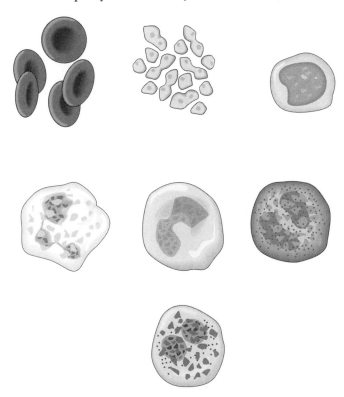

F. CRITICAL THINKING

Answer the following questions in complete sentences.

80. Why is the basement membrane important?

81. Explain the versatility of epithelial tissue.

82. Why is transitional epithelial tissue important?

83. Explain the functions of the mucous membrane.

84. Give an example of a simple and a complex exocrine gland, and state the function of your example.

85. Why would heparin be important to the body?

86. Would an obese person be more or less sensitive to temperature change?

87. How are macrophages a help to the protection of the body?

88. In general, how do muscles work?

89. How will nervous tissue help you pass this course?

90. Why do injuries in older adults heal more slowly?

G. CROSSWORD PUZZLE

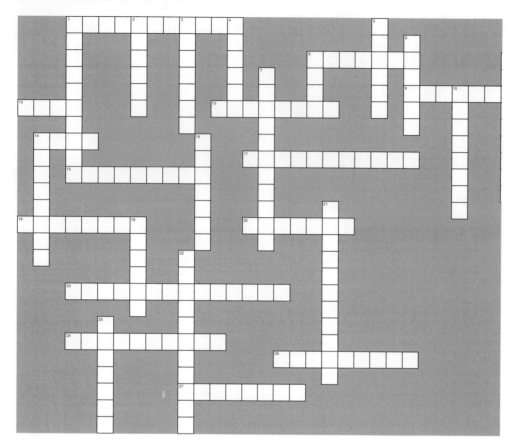

Complete the crossword puzzle using the following clues.

ACROSS

1. Lines circulatory system
8. Fat cells
9. Attach muscle to bone
12. Firm, specialized connective tissue
13. Sweat glands
14. Epithelial tissue protecting underlying tissue
15. Phagocytes in the CNS
17. Wide flat tendon
18. Fiber in matrix
20. Made by mast cells
23. Collagenous fiber in matrix
24. Cells that eat debris
26. Study of tissue
27. Skeletal muscle

DOWN

1. Simple arrangement is one cell thick
2. Groups of cells
3. Cavities in a firm matrix
4. Intercellular material
5. Involuntary muscle tissue
6. Teeth material
7. Motile phagocytes
8. Transmits a nerve impulse
10. Receives and conducts stimuli
11. Produced in response to allergies
12. Flat, irregularly shaped cells
16. Matrix with no visible fibers
19. Nerve cell
21. Forms fibrils
22. Pushes material by muscle contraction
25. Muscle of heart

CHAPTER QUIZ

1. Histology is the study of
   a. cells
   b. organs
   c. tissues
   d. disease
   e. organelles

2. A histiocyte is a cell in
   a. nervous tissue
   b. epithelial tissue
   c. muscle tissue
   d. connective tissue
   e. blood tissue

3. All of the following are functions of epithelial tissue EXCEPT
   a. movement
   b. secretion
   c. protection
   d. excretion
   e. absorption

4. Which tissue has little intercellular material?
   a. loose connective
   b. dense connective
   c. epithelial
   d. specialized connective
   e. none of the above

5. Kupffer's cells are found in the
   a. heart
   b. bladder
   c. liver
   d. teeth
   e. brain

6. Which are cuboidal cells?
   a. pancreas
   b. liver
   c. brain
   d. teeth
   e. ovaries

7. The membrane lining the lungs is the
   a. parietal peritoneum
   b. visceral peritoneum
   c. parietal pleural
   d. visceral pleural
   e. basement

8. The lining of the blood vessels is made up of
   a. cuboidal cells
   b. squamous cells
   c. columnar cells
   d. muscle cells
   e. nervous cells

9. Alveoli of the lungs have which kind of cell arrangement?
   a. psuedostratified
   b. stratified
   c. transitional
   d. simple
   e. common

10. If it is relaxed tissue and the cell layer looks like the teeth of a saw, it is
    a. transitional
    b. stratified
    c. common
    d. psuedostratified
    e. simple

11. Glandular epithelial forms the following type of glands EXCEPT
    a. salivary
    b. sweat
    c. gall
    d. mammary
    e. sebaceous

12. Which glands are unicellular?
    a. tear
    b. endocrine
    c. goblet
    d. simple exocrine
    e. compound exocrine

13. The vessels made up of endothelium made up in a simple cell arrangement are
    a. capillaries
    b. arterioles
    c. arteries
    d. vessels
    e. veins

14. Serous tissue does NOT
    a. protect
    b. excrete
    c. reduce friction
    d. secrete
    e. none of the above

15. Types of connective tissue are cells of the following EXCEPT
    a. loose
    b. areolar
    c. dense
    d. endocardial
    e. specialized

16. A type of loose connective tissue is
    a. tendon
    b. blood
    c. areolar
    d. lymphoid
    e. fibrocartilage

17. The tissue that makes up the subcutaneous layer is
    a. adipose
    b. areolar
    c. hyaline
    d. reticular
    e. specialized

18. Chondrocytes are found in
    a. bone
    b. blood
    c. muscle
    d. cartilage
    e. epithelial

19. The cartilage with tough collagenous fibers is
    a. hyaline
    b. tendons
    c. aponeurosis
    d. fibro
    e. elastic

20. Which of the following is NOT an example of specialized connective tissue?
    a. dentin
    b. fat
    c. bone
    d. blood
    e. lymphoid

21. Kupffer's cells, macrophages and neurolgia make up the
    a. reticuloendothelial system
    b. mast system
    c. lymph system
    d. sensory system
    e. nervous system

22. Synovial membranes line joints and
    a. vessels
    b. bursae
    c. tendons
    d. ligaments
    e. aponeurosis

23. Synovial membranes function in
    a. temperature control
    b. protection from disease
    c. absorption
    d. excretion
    e. friction reduction

24. Which tissue functions as an insulator?
    a. elastic
    b. dense
    c. hyaline
    d. adipose

25. Muscles have the ability to shorten and thicken due to
    a. amine and cytosine
    b. actin and cytosine
    c. hyaline and myosin
    d. actin and myosin
    e. none of the above

26. Of the three muscle types—smooth, striated and cardiac—only striated is
    a. voluntary
    b. involuntary
    c. peristaltic
    d. spindle shape

27. The muscle attached to bones is
    a. smooth
    b. striated
    c. cardiac

28. Intercalated disks are found in which type of muscle?
    a. smooth
    b. striated
    c. cardiac

29. In the nerve cell stimuli are received by the
    a. neuroglia
    b. axon
    c. dendrite
    d. cell body
    e. myelin

30. The supporting cells of the nervous system are the
    a. neuroglia
    b. axon
    c. dendrite
    d. cell body
    e. myelin

CHAPTER 6   THE INTEGUMENTARY SYSTEM

CHAPTER OBJECTIVES

After studying this chapter, you should be able to:

1. Name the layers of the epidermis.
2. Define *keratinization*.
3. Explain why there are skin color differences among people.
4. Describe the anatomic parts of a hair.
5. Compare the two kinds of glands in the skin based on structure and secretion.
6. Explain why sweating is important to survival.
7. Explain how the skin helps regulate body temperature.
8. Name the functions of the skin.

ACTIVITIES

A. COMPLETION

Fill in the blank spaces with the correct term.

1. One of the ways the skin helps regulate body temperature is through the evaporation of _____.

2. The epidermis is a layer of _____ tissue.

3. The second layer is the _____.

4. The dermis is a layer of _____ tissue.

5. The epidermis is composed of _____, _____ and _____ cells.

6. The skin is thickest on the _____ of the hands and the _____ of the feet.

7. As cells move up from the basement membrane, they eventually _____.

8. The protein material of hair and nails is _____.

9. There are _____ layers of the epidermis.

10. Dead cells converted to protein make up the _____ _____.

11. A callus on the foot is called a _____.

12. Cells lose their nuclei and become compact and brittle in the _____.

13. The stratum spinosum contain cells that are _____ in structure.

14. Cells of the epidermis that are capable of dividing are found in the _____ _____.

15. Those cells responsible for skin color are _____.

16. Racial variation in skin color is determined by _____.

17. An absence of melanin produces a condition called _____.

18. True skin is the dermis or _____.

19. A specialist concerned with inflammatory responses of the skin and reactions of the immune system is a/an _____.

20. Besides mammary glands, _____ is a main characteristic of mammals.

21. A bluish tinge to the skin is called _____.

22. Goose bumps are caused by the _____ _____ muscle.

23. Hair growth begins in the _____ _____.

24. A nail will grow from the _____ _____.

25. The eponychium is the _____.

26. _____ is the oily substance responsible for lubrication of the skin and is a product of the _____ _____.

27. The hands and feet are the site of many _____ _____.

28. Sweating causes odor because of _____ activity.

29. Sensations recorded by the skin are _____ and _____.

30. Inhibition of water loss by the skin is due to its _____ content.

31. A common chronic skin disorder is _____.

32. Herpes simplex causes _____ _____.

33. The varicella (chickenpox) virus is responsible for _____.

34. Sweat glands are activated by _____.

35. A patchy skin disease is _____.

B. MATCHING

Match the term on the right with the definition on the left.

36. _____ skin modifications

37. _____ epidermal cellular links

38. _____ clear layer

39. _____ varies skin pigmentation

40. _____ affected by first-degree burns

41. _____ subcutaneous layer

42. _____ hair's principal portion

43. _____ hair's visible portion

44. _____ hair texture

45. _____ visible nail

46. _____ oily gland

47. _____ salty liquid secretion

48. _____ skin function

49. _____ skin cancer

50. _____ human papillomavirus

a. epidermis

b. shaft

c. sweat

d. keratin

e. appendages

f. warts

g. nail body

h. desmosomes

i. hypodermis

j. melanin

k. melanoma

l. stratum lucidum

m. cortex

n. thermoregulation

o. sebaceous

C. KEY TERMS

Use the text to look up the following terms. Write the definition or explanation.

51. Basal cell carcinoma: _____

_____

52. Callus: _____

_____

53. Cortex: _____

_____

54. Desmosome: _____

_____

55. Hair follicle: _____

_____

56. Keratinization: _____

_____

57. Lunula: _____

_____

58. Medulla: _____

_____

59. Papillary portion: _____

_____

60. Partial-thickness burns: _____

_____

61. Reticular portion: _____

_____

62. Second-degree burns: _____

_____

63. Squamous cell carcinoma: _____

_____

64. Strata: _____

_____

65. Stratum basale: _____

_____

D. LABELING EXERCISE

66. Label the parts of the skin as indicated in Figure 6-1.

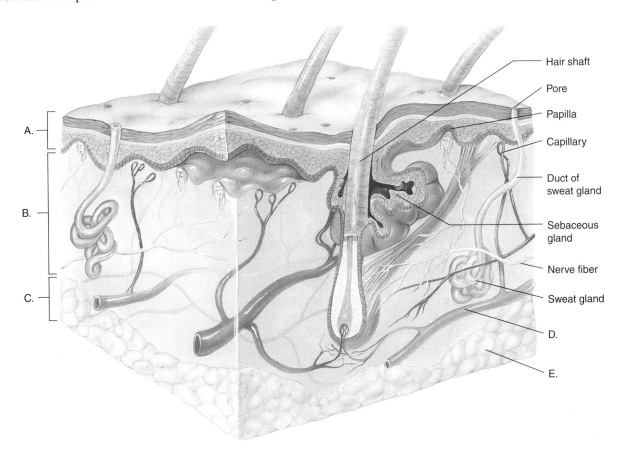

a. _____

b. _____

c. _____

d. _____

e. _____

67. Label the parts of the hair as indicated in Figure 6-2.

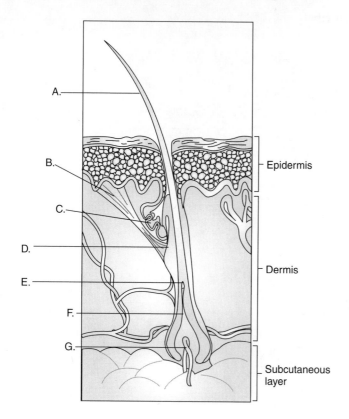

a. _____

b. _____

c. _____

d. _____

e. _____

f. _____

g. _____

E. COLORING EXERCISE

68. Using Figure 6-3, color the matrix red, cuticle brown and nail blue.

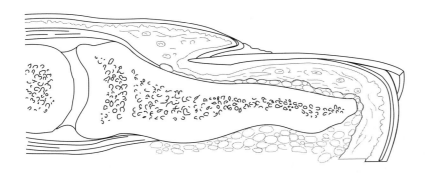

F. CRITICAL THINKING

Answer the following questions in complete sentences.

69. How does the stratum corneum protect against disease?

70. Why is the stratum germinativum so important?

71. Why are third-degree burns so traumatic?

72. Why is the dermis called the true skin?

73. Why would deep tissue trauma cause hair loss?

74. If a nail is completely torn out, why does it grow back?

75. Explain why adolescents experience more acne than adults.

76. Is the sweat gland an exocrine or endocrine gland?

77. Why are sports drinks so important to athletes?

78. How can impetigo cause other diseases?

79. Is ringworm a correct term for the disease?

80. What changes occur in the integumentary system as the body ages?

G. CROSSWORD PUZZLE

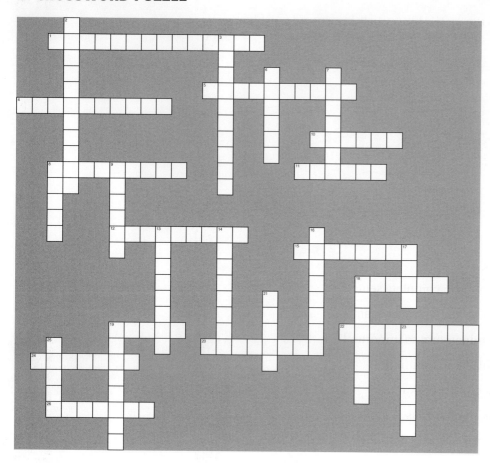

Complete the crossword puzzle using the following clues.

ACROSS

1. Skin cell process
4. Subcutaneous tissue
5. Cellular links
8. Oily glands
10. Distinctive layers
11. White crescent of the nail
12. Outer layer of skin
15. Fungus-caused skin disease
18. Thickened skin area
19. Visible part of hair
20. Bacteria-caused skin disease
22. System that secretes hormones
24. Skin pigmentation
26. Middle part of hair

DOWN

2. Produces skin color
3. Means a covering
6. True skin
7. Protein material
8. Cools skin
9. Principal portion of hair
13. Shedding scalp cells
14. Absence of skin color
16. Irregular patches of skin pigmentation
17. Groupings of melanocytes
18. Bluish skin discoloration
19. Disease caused by the chickenpox virus
21. Caused by human papillomavirus
23. Eponychium
25. Oil for skin lubrication

CHAPTER QUIZ

1. A bony prominence on the foot receiving excess friction may develop a
   a. callus
   b. wart
   c. blackhead
   d. corn
   e. none of the above

2. Albinism is caused by a lack of
   a. desmosome
   b. osteocytes
   c. melanocytes
   d. mast cells
   e. none of the above

3. Excessive production of sebum may cause
   a. psoriasis
   b. callus
   c. corns
   d. shingles
   e. none of the above

4. Kerinatinized cells contain no
   a. nucleus
   b. cell wall
   c. fluid
   d. cell membrane
   e. none of the above

5. Flexibility, entirety and whole continuous structure are qualities of the skin due to
   a. a callus
   b. desmosomes
   c. melanocytes
   d. osteocytes
   e. corns

6. The layer of the epidermis in which mitosis takes place is the stratum
   a. spinosum
   b. granulosum
   c. germinativum
   d. corneum
   e. lucidum

7. A lipid covering of cells is found in the stratum
   a. spinosum
   b. granulosum
   c. germinativum
   d. corneum
   e. lucidum

8. Cells of the stratum corneum contain as many as
   a. 10 layers
   b. 5 layers
   c. 20 layers
   d. 25 layers
   e. none of the above

9. Stratum basale is found in the stratum
   a. spinosum
   b. granulosum
   c. germinativum
   d. corneum
   e. lucidum

10. Racial color differences are a result of variation in quantity of
    a. astrocytes
    b. desmosome
    c. melanocytes
    d. karocytes
    e. none of the above

11. True skin contains which of the following?
    a. papillary portion
    b. hypodermis
    c. areolar tissue
    d. adipose tissue
    e. none of the above

12. A bluish tinge of the skin is called
    a. psoriasis
    b. cyanosis
    c. shingles
    d. ringworm
    e. none of the above

13. Besides hair, another main characteristic of mammals is
    a. sweat glands
    b. ceruminous glands
    c. mammary glands
    d. adrenal glands
    e. none of the above

14. Hair covers all of the body EXCEPT the
    a. arms
    b. legs
    c. face
    d. genitalia
    e. none of the above

15. Arrector pili muscles engage when we get
    a. a chill
    b. psoriasis
    c. papilloma virus
    d. shingles
    e. cold sores

16. Texture of hair is a result of
    a. melanocytes
    b. astrocytes
    c. desmosomes
    d. melanin
    e. keratin

17. A white crescent located at the proximal end of the nail is the
    a. nail bed
    b. lunula
    c. cuticle
    d. root
    e. none of the above

18. Another name for the eponychium is
    a. cuticle
    b. nail body
    c. nail bed
    d. lunula
    e. nail root

19. Shiny hair is a result of
    a. melanocytes
    b. sebum
    c. sweat
    d. callus
    e. cerumen

20. Sebaceous secretion is controlled by the
    a. exocrine system
    b. lymph system
    c. endocrine system
    d. circulatory system
    e. none of the above

21. Besides fatty oils, blackheads are produced in the presence of
    a. water
    b. heat
    c. cold
    d. air
    e. none of the above

22. Sweat odor is caused by
    a. melanocytes
    b. astrocytes
    c. desmosomes
    d. bacteria
    e. yeast

23. External environmental changes are registered by receptor sites; these changes are
    a. wet and dry
    b. temperature and moisture
    c. pressure and moisture
    d. temperature and pressure
    e. none of the above

24. Which of the following are NOT protective functions?
    a. sunlight
    b. bacteria
    c. some chemical agents
    d. water loss
    e. organic pesticides

25. Temperature regulation is critical due to excessive heat affecting
    a. enzymes
    b. blood
    c. urea
    d. sugar
    e. water

26. A condition characterized by baldness that is influenced by genetic factors, hormones, malnutrition, diabetes, drug interactions and/or chemotherapy is
    a. molds
    b. alopecia
    c. psoriasis
    d. vitiligo
    e. impetigo

27. The skin is involved in the production of
    a. ATP
    b. phosphate
    c. calcium
    d. vitamin D
    e. none of the above

28. The most dangerous type of skin cancer is
    a. malignant melanoma
    b. basal cell carcinoma
    c. squamous cell carcinoma
    d. none of the above

29. A children's disease that can cause a related disease in adults is
    a. ringworm
    b. chickenpox
    c. psoriasis
    d. impetigo
    e. none of the above

30. The herpes simplex virus causes
    a. warts
    b. impetigo
    c. shingles
    d. cold sores
    e. psoriasis

CHAPTER 7   THE SKELETAL SYSTEM

CHAPTER OBJECTIVES

After studying this chapter, you should be able to:

1. Name the functions of the skeletal system.
2. Name the two types of ossification.
3. Describe why diet can affect bone development in children and bone maintenance in older adults.
4. Describe the histology of compact bone.
5. Define and give examples of bone markings.
6. Name the cranial and facial bones.
7. Name the bones of the axial and appendicular skeleton.

ACTIVITIES

A. COMPLETION

Fill in the blank spaces with the correct term.

1. The five functions of the skeletal system include _____, _____, _____, _____ and _____ _____.

2. Osteoblasts invade _____ and begin the process of ossification.

3. The _____ is a fibrovascular membrane that covers bone; the _____ is the membrane that lines the medullary cavity.

4. Bone remodeling is made possible by _____ and _____.

5. The process of ossification can be either _____ or _____.

6. Correct calcium ion concentration in blood and bone is maintained by _____ and _____.

7. _____ bone is dense and strong, whereas _____ bone is spongy.

8. An osteon, also called the _____ _____, allows for the effective metabolism of bone cells.

9. The spaces within cancellous bone contain _____ _____ _____, which is responsible for hematopoiesis.

10. Long bones consist of a _____, _____ and a(an) _____.

11. _____ bones are enclosed in a tendon and fascial tissue.

12. An obvious bony prominence is called a(an) _____.

13. A depression or cavity in or on a bone is called a(an) _____.

14. The skeleton is divided into two main parts, the _____ and the _____.

15. The _____ bone is a single bone that forms the posterior base of the cranium.

16. The anchor bone for the cranium is the _____ _____ _____.

17. The freely movable bone of the face is the _____ _____.

18. The spinal cord passes through a space called the _____ _____.

19. The largest and strongest vertebrae are those of the _____ section of the spine.

20. _____ are the bones of the fingers and toes.

B. MATCHING

Match the term on the right with the definition on the left.

21. _____ result of abnormal endochondral ossification at the epiphyseal plate of long bones

    a. osteoporosis

22. _____ lateral curvature of the spine

    b. lordosis

23. _____ the laminae of the posterior vertebral arch do not unite at the midline

    c. giantism

24. _____ disorder characterized by disease in bone mass with increased susceptibility to fractures

    d. axis

25. _____ rupture of fibrocartilage surrounding an intervertebral disk

    e. kyphosis

26. _____ irregular thickening and softening of the bones with excessive bone destruction

    f. scoliosis

27. _____ swayback

    g. false ribs

28. _____ strongest portion of the hip bone

    h. spina bifida

29. _____ accentuated curvature of the spine in the upper thoracic region

    i. herniated disk

30. _____ second vertebra

    j. incus

31. _____ direct articulation with the sternum

    k. patella

32. _____ indirect articulation with the sternum

    l. carpals

33. _____ do not attach anteriorly

    m. ischium

34. _____ bones of the wrist

    n. true ribs

35. _____ anvil

    o. hyoid

36. _____ kneecap

    p. osteoprogenitor

37. _____ give rise to osteoblasts

    q. Paget's disease

38. _____ immovable joint line of the cranium

    r. floating ribs

39. _____ tie bone to bones

    s. suture

40. _____ tongue attached to it

    t. ligaments

C. KEY TERMS

Use the text to look up the following terms. Write the definition or explanation.

41. Acetabulum: _____

_____

42. Acromial process: _____

_____

43. Calcaneus: _____

_____

44. Capitate: _____

_____

45. Cervical vertebrae: _____

_____

46. Condyle: _____

_____

47. Coracoid process: _____

_____

48. Fontanelle: _____

_____

49. Foramen: _____

_____

50. Gladiolus: _____

_____

51. Hamate: _____

_____

52. Haversian (system): _____

_____

53. Hematopoiesis: _____

_____

54. Lunate: _____

_____

55. Malleus: _____

_____

56. Manubrium: _____

_____

57. Meatus: _____

_____

58. Obturator foramen: _____

_____

59. Ossification: _____

_____

60. Osteomalacia: _____

_____

61. Osteon: _____

_____

62. Phalanx: _____

_____

63. Pisiform: _____

_____

64. Sagittal suture: _____

_____

65. Stapes: _____

_____

66. Talus: _____

_____

67. Trabeculae: _____

_____

68. Triquetral: _____

_____

69. Tympanic plate: _____

_____

70. Vomer (bone): _____

_____

71. Xiphoid: _____

_____

72. Zygomatic (bones): _____

_____

D. LABELING EXERCISE

73. Label the bones of the skeletal system as indicated in Figure 7-1.

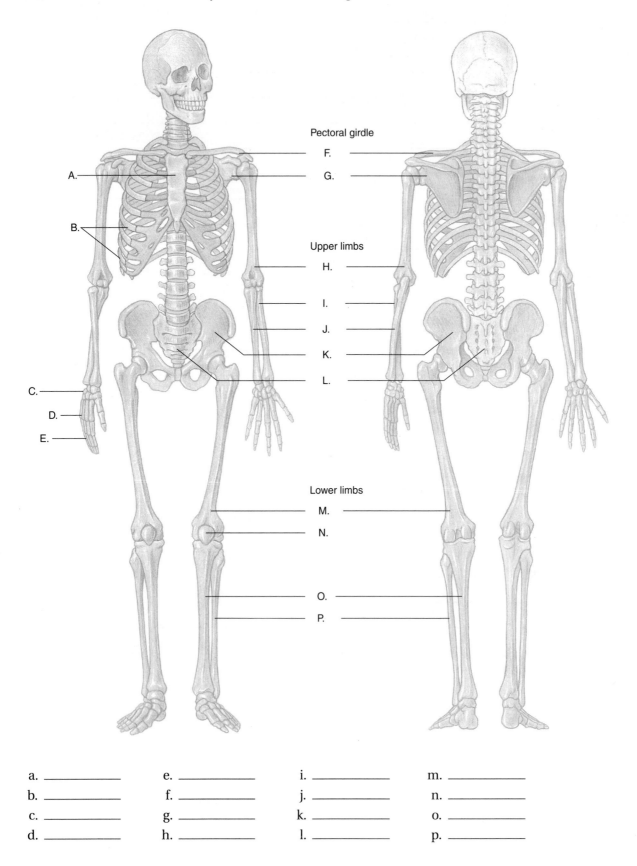

Pectoral girdle
F.
G.

A.

B.

Upper limbs
H.
I.
J.
K.
L.

C.
D.
E.

Lower limbs
M.
N.

O.
P.

a. _____   e. _____   i. _____   m. _____
b. _____   f. _____   j. _____   n. _____
c. _____   g. _____   k. _____   o. _____
d. _____   h. _____   l. _____   p. _____

74. Label the parts of the spinal column as indicated in Figure 7-2.

A. C_1 _____

B. C_2 _____

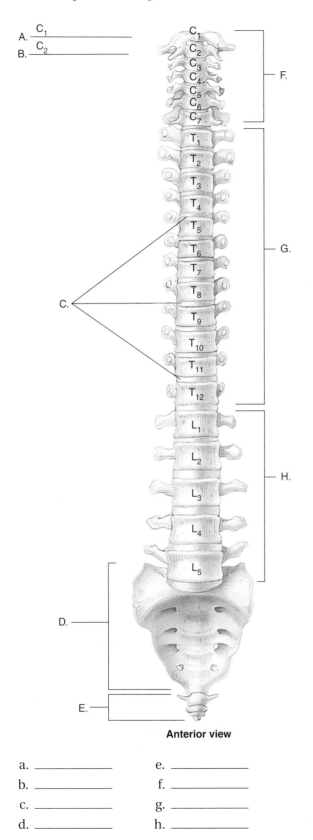

Anterior view

a. _____   e. _____

b. _____   f. _____

c. _____   g. _____

d. _____   h. _____

75. Label the bones of the thoracic cage as indicated in Figure 7-3.

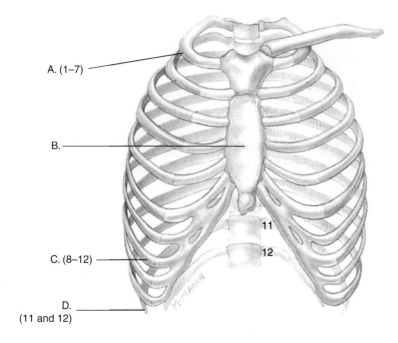

A. (1–7)

B.

11

12

C. (8–12)

D.
(11 and 12)

a. _____
b. _____
c. _____
d. _____

76. Label the bones of the hand and wrist as indicated in Figure 7-4.

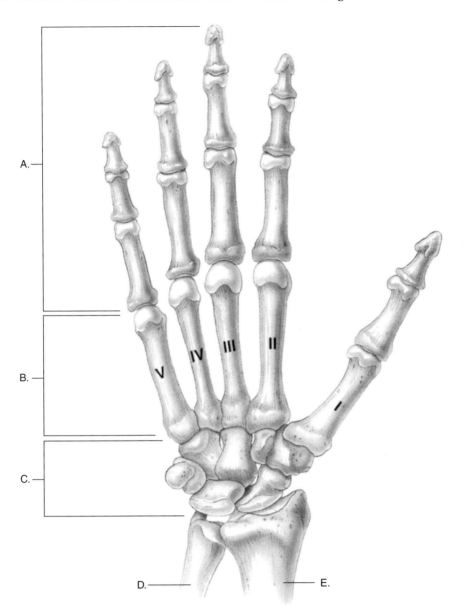

a. _____
b. _____
c. _____
d. _____
e. _____

77. Label the bones of the foot as indicated in Figure 7-5.

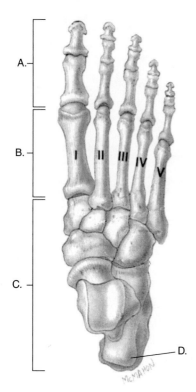

a. _____

b. _____

c. _____

d. _____

E. COLORING EXERCISE

78. Using Figure 7-6, color the skull blue, the axial skeleton green and the appendicular skeleton red.

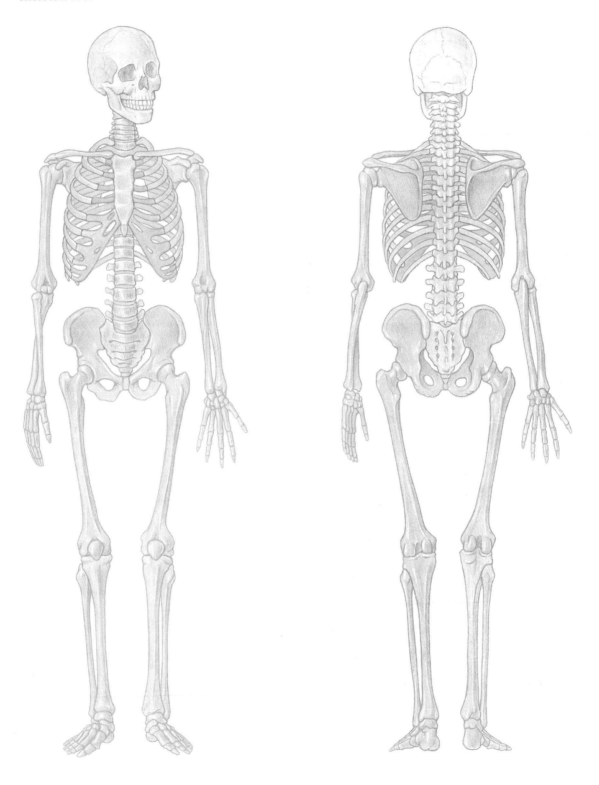

F. CRITICAL THINKING

Answer the following questions in complete sentences.

79. Why is the calcaneus a large strong bone?

80. Differentiate osteoblast, osteoclast and osteoprogenitor cell.

81. How does the body maintain proper calcium balance?

82. Differentiate red and yellow bone marrow.

83. What defect results from fusion failure of the maxillary bones? Why would it affect speech?

84. Why are the 11th and 12th pairs of ribs called "floating ribs"?

85. The glenoid fossa is similar to what structure of the hip?

86. Why is rickets a common disease in many third world countries?

87. Differentiate between tendon and ligament.

88. Explain how aging affects bone and its supporting tissues.

89. Identify the skeletal system career option that would best fit your interests and explain why.

90. Briefly explain the difference among an orthotist, an orthopedist and a prosthetist.

91. Describe what a Doctor of Chiropractic, or chiropractor, does and the training required to become one.

G. CROSSWORD PUZZLE

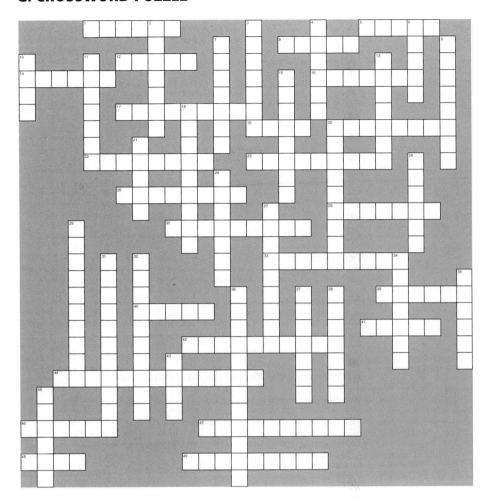

Complete the crossword puzzle using the following clues.

ACROSS

1. Narrow junction between two bones
5. Sharp, slender projection
8. Bone supporting the tongue
12. Ear bone referred to as the anvil
14. Five unfused vertabrae in the lower back
16. Shoulder blade
17. Mature osteoblast
19. Connects the head to the rest of a long bone
20. 12 vertabrae that connect with the ribs
22. Small rounded bone

DOWN

2. Disease caused by lack of vitamin D
3. Opening in bone for nerve or blood vessel, etc.
4. Bone depressions
6. Bones forming the bridge of the nose
7. Knuckle-like prominence at an articulation point
9. Small, rounded process
10. Bone type that protects vital body parts
11. Ear bone referred to as the hammer
13. Longest bone of the upper arm
15. Pulley-shaped process

ACROSS

23. Perforating canals
26. Bones that make up part of the orbit of the inner angle of the eye
28. Forms the dense, outer layer of bone
30. Part of the sternum resembling the handle of a sword
33. Finger bones
39. Long, tubelike passage
40. Narrow ridge of bone
41. Cavity within a bone
42. Fibrovascular membrane covering a bone
44. Making blood cells
46. Shorter bone of the forearm
47. Flared portion at the ends of a long bone
48. Terminal enlargement of a bone
49. Lines the medullary cavity of long bones

DOWN

18. Single bone forming the back of the cranium
20. Meshwork of interconnecting bone sections
21. Zygomatic bone
24. Furrow or groove
25. Tiny cavities between lamellae
27. Shaft of long bone
29. Soft spot on a baby's head
31. Cells responsible for reabsorption of bone
32. Spongy bone
34. Breastbone
35. Haversian canal
36. Formation of bone by osteoblasts
37. Ring of bone around the haversian canal
38. Bone supporting the nasal cavity structure
43. Bone whose length exceeds its width
45. Ear bone referred to as the stirrup

CHAPTER QUIZ

1. Which of the following is NOT a function of the skeletal system?
   a. support
   b. protection
   c. nutrient absorption
   d. movement
   e. storage of mineral salts

2. Longitudinal growth of bone continues until approximately what age in boys?
   a. 15
   b. 13
   c. 14
   d. 21
   e. 16

3. Undifferentiated bone cells are called
   a. osteoclasts
   b. osteoprogenitors
   c. osteoblasts
   d. osteons
   e. osteocytes

4. The skeletal system is most closely associated with which system?
   a. respiratory
   b. digestive
   c. excretory
   d. muscular
   e. lymphatic

5. The hormones responsible for proper calcium balance in the body are
   a. calcitonin/potassium
   b. thyroxine/calcitonin
   c. renin/parathormone
   d. parathormone/calcitonin
   e. progesterone/epinephrine

6. Osteomalacia in adults is known as what disease in children?
   a. measles
   b. spina bifida
   c. Paget's disease
   d. rickets
   e. Graves' disease

7. Hematopoiesis takes place in which type of bone?
   a. compact
   b. flat
   c. hard
   d. short
   e. cancellous

8. The haversian system is necessary for
   a. maintaining calcium balance
   b. hematopoiesis
   c. protection of soft tissue
   d. ossification
   e. effective metabolism of bone cells

9. Blood cells in all stages of development are found in
   a. lacunae
   b. canaliculi
   c. yellow marrow
   d. red marrow
   e. Volkmann's canals

10. Bones can be divided into how many categories?
    a. 5
    b. 7
    c. 2
    d. 10
    e. 3

11. Long bones have a shaft called a(n)
    a. epiphysis
    b. diaphysis
    c. metaphysis
    d. osteon
    e. medullary

12. The medullary shaft is filled with
    a. blood
    b. yellow marrow
    c. red marrow
    d. cartilage
    e. trabeculae

13. Examples of flat bones are
    a. wrist/ankle
    b. ribs/scapula
    c. tibia/fibula
    d. carpal/tarsal
    e. vertebrae/auditory ossicles

14. A sesamoid bone is the
    a. patella
    b. sternum
    c. clavicle
    d. phalanges
    e. mandible

15. Which of the following is NOT a process?
    a. meatus
    b. condyle
    c. tubercle
    d. crest
    e. trochlea

16. Which of the following is NOT a fossa?
    a. suture
    b. sinus
    c. trochanter
    d. sulcus
    e. foramen

17. Which two bones form the upper sides and roof of the cranium?
    a. occipital
    b. frontal
    c. parietal
    d. temporal
    e. sphenoid

18. The cheekbones are which bones?
    a. nasal
    b. palatine
    c. malar
    d. lacrimal
    e. turbinates

19. Bones act as storage areas for mineral salts and
    a. muscle tissue
    b. blood
    c. fats
    d. lymph
    e. waste

20. Which bone of the axial skeleton has no articulation with other bones?
    a. vomer
    b. temporal
    c. hyoid
    d. palatine
    e. occipital

21. There are how many sections of the spine?
    a. 4
    b. 15
    c. 7
    d. 5
    e. 10

22. The two sections of the spine that consist of fused bones are the
    a. cervical/coccygeal
    b. thoracic/sacrum
    c. lumbar/cervical
    d. sacrum/lumbar
    e. coccygeal/sacrum

23. Abnormal curvature of the spine in the lumbar region is known as swayback or
    a. kyphosis
    b. rickets
    c. osteoporosis
    d. Paget's disease
    e. lordosis

24. The manubrium articulates with the
    a. scapula
    b. axis
    c. sacrum
    d. acromion process
    e. clavicle

25. The lower five pairs of ribs are called
    a. true ribs
    b. floating ribs
    c. false ribs
    d. costal ribs
    e. paired ribs

26. Two bony projections of the scapula are called the
    a. acromial processes
    b. glenoid processes
    c. coracoid processes
    d. acetabulum
    e. spinous processes

27. The longer bone of the forearm is the
    a. humerus
    b. radius
    c. ulna
    d. scaphoid
    e. carpal

28. The coxal bones make up the
    a. pubis
    b. ischium
    c. ilium
    d. acetabulum
    e. pelvic girdle

29. The longest and heaviest bone of the body is the
    a. ilium
    b. tibia
    c. humerus
    d. patella
    e. femur

30. The shinbone is the
    a. tibia
    b. fibula
    c. calcaneus
    d. patella
    e. femur

31. Which of the foot bones is the largest?
    a. cuboid
    b. phalanges
    c. calcaneus
    d. navicular
    e. talus

32. Decreased height of the longitudinal arches is known as
    a. rickets
    b. Graves' disease
    c. kyphosis
    d. tinea pedis
    e. pes planus

33. Which of the following is NOT a bone of the axial skeleton?
    a. sternum
    b. occipital
    c. xiphoid
    d. radius
    e. coccyx

34. Which of the following is NOT a bone of the appendicular skeleton?
    a. ulna
    b. ribs
    c. femur
    d. patella
    e. calcaneus

35. Which of the following attaches bone to bone?
    a. tendons
    b. aponeurosis
    c. ligament
    d. muscle
    e. none of the above

CHAPTER 8   THE ARTICULAR SYSTEM

CHAPTER OBJECTIVES

After studying this chapter, you should be able to:

1. Name and describe the three types of joints.
2. Name the two types of synarthroses joints.
3. Name examples of the two types of amphiarthroses joints.
4. Name and give examples of the six types of diarthroses or synovial joints.
5. Describe the capsular nature of a synovial joint.
6. Describe the three types of bursae.
7. Name some of the disorders of joints.
8. Describe the possible movements at synovial joints.

ACTIVITIES

A. COMPLETION

Fill in the blank spaces with the correct term.

1. A union between two or more bones is a _____.
2. Joints are classified by _____ and _____.
3. Skull joints are called _____.
4. Besides sutures, there are two other types of synarthroses; they are _____ and _____.
5. Those joints allowing only slight movement are _____.
6. A joint in which two bony surfaces are connected by hyaline cartilage is a _____.
7. Synovial joints are also called _____.
8. Synovial joints are characterized by the presence of a _____ and a _____.
9. A diarthrosis joint provides a smooth gliding surface because of _____.
10. A buffer between two weight-bearing bones is provided by _____.
11. The joint providing the greatest range of motion in the body is found in the _____.
12. Functions of the synovial joints include _____, _____ and _____.
13. A decrease in the angle of a joint is denoted as _____.
14. If a joint is forced beyond its normal range of extension, it is _____.
15. Movement of a limb away from the midline of the body is _____.
16. Moving a limb in a direction that causes the bone to describe a cone is _____.
17. _____ is a movement placing the palm in an anterior position.
18. Moving the palm of the hand so that it faces down is called _____.
19. Move the body forward for _____ and backward for _____.

20. _____ is raising the body.

21. Only primates can perform the movement called _____.

22. A ball-and-socket joint will have a ball-shaped head fitting into a _____ _____.

23. In the joint of the hip, the ball-shaped head of the femur fits into the _____.

24. An example of a hinge joint is the _____.

25. A condyloid joint is also known as an _____ joint.

26. The thumb is an example of a _____ joint.

27. Gliding joints are found in the _____.

28. Closed sacs with a synovial lining are _____.

29. Inflammation of a joint is called _____.

30. Degenerative joint disease is sometimes known as _____.

B. MATCHING

Match the term on the right with the definition on the left.

31. _____ accumulation of uric acid crystals

32. _____ rheumatism

33. _____ connective tissue disorder

34. _____ inflammation of synovial bursa

35. _____ bacterial infection

36. _____ one tendon overlies another

37. _____ subfascial bursae

38. _____ example, atlas vertebra

39. _____ lowering part of the body

40. _____ move the sole outward

41. _____ increase joint angle

42. _____ move around the central axis

43. _____ pushing the foot up

44. _____ move the limb toward the midline

45. _____ reinforce a joint capsule

a. depression

b. pivot joint

c. extension

d. gout

e. primary fibrositis

f. adduction

g. ligaments

h. between muscles

i. bursitis

j. dorsiflexion

k. rheumatoid arthritis

l. rotation

m. eversion

n. rheumatic fever

o. subtendinous bursae

C. KEY TERMS

Use the text to look up the following terms. Write the definition or explanation.

46. Abduction: _____

_____

47. Adduction: _____

_____

48. Amphiarthrosis: _____

_____

49. Bursae: _____

_____

50. Condyloid joint: _____

_____

51. Dorsiflexion: _____

_____

52. Eversion: _____

_____

53. Fascia: _____

_____

54. Gliding joint: _____

_____

55. Osteoarthritis: _____

_____

56. Primary fibrositis: _____

_____

57. Reposition: _____

_____

58. Subcutaneous bursae: _____

_____

59. Subtendinous bursae: _____

_____

60. Symphysis: _____

_____

D. LABELING EXERCISE

61. Label the joints as indicated in Figure 8-1.

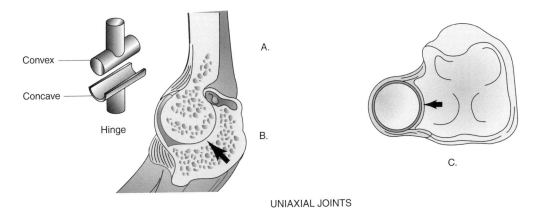

UNIAXIAL JOINTS

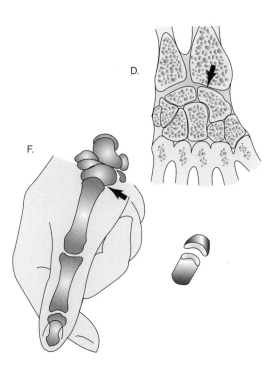

BIAXIAL JOINTS

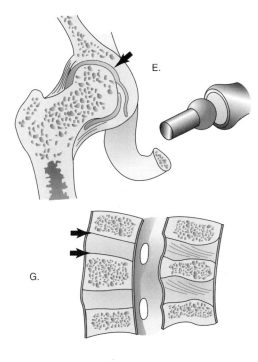

MULTIAXIAL JOINTS

a. _____

b. _____

c. _____

d. _____

e. _____

f. _____

g. _____

62. Label the parts of the knee joint as indicated in Figure 8-2.

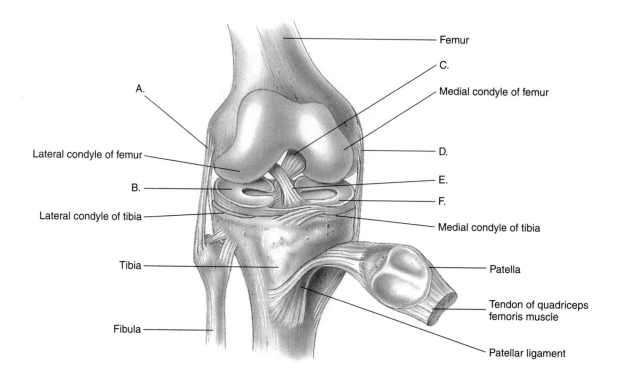

Femur

C.

Medial condyle of femur

A.

Lateral condyle of femur

D.

B.

E.

F.

Lateral condyle of tibia

Medial condyle of tibia

Tibia

Patella

Tendon of quadriceps femoris muscle

Fibula

Patellar ligament

a. _____

b. _____

c. _____

d. _____

e. _____

f. _____

E. COLORING EXERCISE

63. Using Figure 8-3, color the bones red, the articular cartilage blue, the synovial membrane green and the synovial fluid yellow.

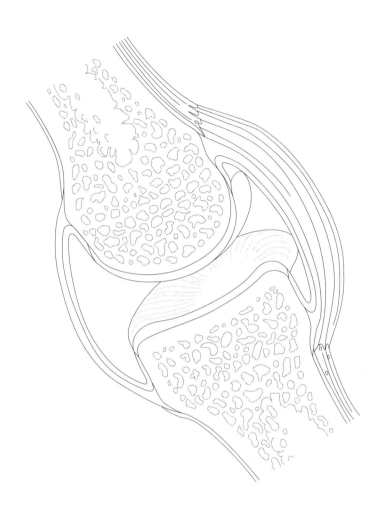

F. CRITICAL THINKING

Answer the following questions in complete sentences.

64. What are the criteria for classifying joints?

65. Why do some authors consider syndesmosis an example of amphiarthrosis?

66. Differentiate amphiarthrosis and diarthrosis.

67. Why does the shoulder joint have the greatest range of motion?

68. Why is moderate, regular exercise important as we age?

69. Why are primates the only animals to use hand tools?

70. What is meant by uniaxial, biaxial, and multiaxial?

71. Of the three types of bursae, which would be least likely to have bursitis? Explain.

72. Why would rheumatic fever affect the heart?

G. CROSSWORD PUZZLE

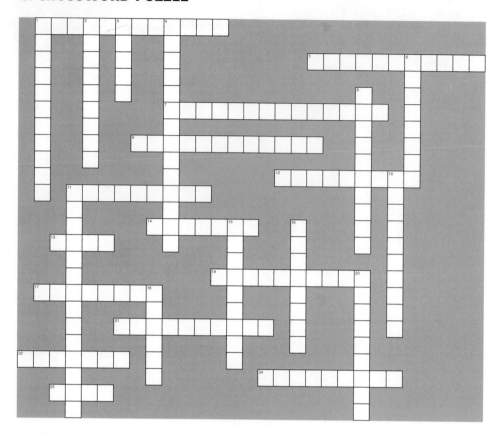

Complete the crossword puzzle using the following clues.

ACROSS

1. Immovable joint
5. Synovial joints
7. Joints with slight movement
9. Joint
11. Palm down
12. Sole in
13. Hinge joint
14. Condyloid joint
17. Inflamed bursa
19. Ball and socket joint
21. Move a part backward
22. Decreasing the angle between joints
23. Excessive uric acid
24. Buffer between vertebrae

DOWN

1. Bones move as one
2. Inflamed joint
3. Saddle joint
4. Degenerative joint disease
6. Around an axis
8. Lower a part
10. Motion unique to the thumb
11. Foot pushes down
15. Toward the midline
16. Bone-to-bone connector
18. Joints of skull
20. Synovial fluid

CHAPTER QUIZ

1. Joints are classified into how many major groups?

   a. 1

   b. 2

   c. 3

   d. 4

   e. 5

2. In a suture, the bones are united by

   a. ligaments

   b. tendons

   c. epithelial tissue

   d. adipose tissue

   e. fibrous tissue

3. In a syndesmosis joint, the bursae are united by

   a. ligaments

   b. tendons

   c. epithelial tissue

   d. adipose tissue

   e. fibrous tissue

4. A tooth is an example of a(n)

   a. synchondrosis

   b. diarthrosis

   c. amphiarthrosis

   d. gomphosis

   e. symphysis

5. A joint in which the bones are connected by a disk of fibrocartilage is a

   a. synchondrosis

   b. diarthrosis

   c. synarthrosis

   d. gomphosis

   e. symphysis

6. Two bony surfaces are connected by hyaline cartilage; this is a

   a. synchondrosis

   b. diarthrosis

   c. synarthrosis

   d. gomphosis

   e. symphysis

7. Cartilage supplying a smooth, gliding surface is

   a. fibrous

   b. aponeurosis

   c. articular

   d. hyaline

   e. collagenous

8. Material connecting one bone to another and forming a joint capsule is
   a. ligamentous
   b. collagenous
   c. tendinous
   d. adipose
   e. cartilagineous

9. The femur joins with the tibia at its distal end and fits into what at its proximal end?
   a. glenoid fossa
   b. symphysis
   c. carpal
   d. acetabulum
   e. none of the above

10. The proximal end of the femur is attached at the joint by
    a. tendons
    b. ligaments
    c. cartilage
    d. collagen
    e. none of the above

11. Which of the following movements is possible in a synarthrosis joint?
    a. flexion
    b. rotation
    c. abduction
    d. opposition
    e. none of the above

12. With circumduction, the bone movement is a circle and a(n)
    a. square
    b. extension
    c. cone
    d. rotation
    e. none of the above

13. The opposite of abduction is
    a. circumduction
    b. adduction
    c. flexion
    d. dorsiflexion
    e. none of the above

14. The opposite of dorsiflexion is
    a. extension
    b. adduction
    c. inversion
    d. plantar flexion
    e. none of the above

15. Supination and pronation refer to movement of the
    a. foot and ankle
    b. knee and hip
    c. wrist and elbow
    d. none of the above

16. If the palm is moved from posterior to anterior, this is an example of
    a. inversion
    b. supination
    c. pronation
    d. rotation
    e. none of the above

17. Opposition is unique to
    a. primates
    b. man
    c. mammals
    d. apes
    e. none of the above

18. The number of diarthroses or synovial joints is
    a. 2
    b. 4
    c. 6
    d. 8
    e. none of the above

19. A convex surface fits into a concave surface. What kind of joint is this?
    a. hinge
    b. condyloid
    c. pivot
    d. saddle
    e. gliding

20. An ellipsoidal joint is also known as which type of joint?
    a. hinge
    b. condyloid
    c. pivot
    d. saddle
    e. gliding

21. The type of joint formed by opposing planes surfaces is a
    a. hinge
    b. condyloid
    c. pivot
    d. saddle
    e. gliding

22. The joint allowing for thumb opposition is the
    a. hinge
    b. condyloid
    c. pivot
    d. saddle
    e. gliding

23. Subfascial bursae are located between
    a. bones
    b. muscles
    c. ligaments
    d. tendon
    e. skin and bone

24. Subcutaneous bursae are found between
    a. bones
    b. muscles
    c. ligaments
    d. tendons
    e. skin and bone

25. Subtendinous bursae are found between
    a. bones
    b. muscles
    c. ligaments
    d. tendons
    e. skin and bone

26. Synovial sac inflammation is
    a. bursitis
    b. arthritis
    c. osteoarthritis
    d. gout
    e. primary fibrositis

27. Total joint inflammation is
    a. bursitis
    b. arthritis
    c. osteoarthritis
    d. gout
    e. primary fibrositis

28. Lumbago is
    a. bursitis
    b. arthritis
    c. osteoarthritis
    d. gout
    e. primary fibrositis

29. Which of the following causes joint degeneration?
    a. bursitis
    b. arthritis
    c. osteoarthritis
    d. gout
    e. primary fibrositis

30. Which of the following can cause kidney damage?
    a. bursitis
    b. arthritis
    c. osteoarthritis
    d. gout
    e. primary fibrositi

CHAPTER 9   THE MUSCULAR SYSTEM

CHAPTER OBJECTIVES

After studying this chapter, you should be able to:

1. Describe the gross and microscopic anatomy of skeletal muscle.
2. Describe and compare the basic differences between the anatomy of skeletal, smooth and cardiac muscle.
3. Explain the current concept of muscle contraction based on three factors: neuroelectrical, chemical and energy sources.
4. Define *muscle tone* and compare isotonic and isometric contractions.
5. List factors that can cause muscles to malfunction, causing various disorders.
6. Name and identify the location of major superficial muscles of the body.

ACTIVITIES

A. COMPLETION

Fill in the blank spaces with the correct term.

1. Skeletal muscle is striated and _____.

2. Because their length is greater than their width, skeletal muscle cells are referred to as muscle _____.

3. The sarcolemma is surrounded by three types of connective tissue; they are the _____, the _____ and the _____.

4. A bands are the _____ bands and I bands are the _____ bands.

5. There are no cross-bridges in the _____.

6. The actual process of contraction occurs in the area called the _____.

7. Muscle fibrils are surrounded by membranes in the form of _____ and _____.

8. These structures are referred to as the _____ system.

9. An irregular curtain around each of the fibrils is the _____ _____.

10. A motor unit is innervated by a _____ _____.

11. Each motor unit in the _____ muscle contains about 10 muscle cells.

12. A muscle fiber's membrane is surrounded by _____.

13. The two minerals causing a resting potential in a muscle are _____ and _____.

14. The electrical potential is caused by a rapid influx of _____ ions.

15. A muscle cell generating its own impulse is called its _____ _____.

16. The two inhibitor substances surrounding the actin are _____ and _____.

17. The substance negating their effect is _____.

18. The discoverer of the protein myosin was _____.

19. During contraction, the width of the A bands remains constant while the _____ move closer.

20. The four sources of ATP for the energy of contraction are _____, _____, _____ _____ _____ and _____ plus two ATP.

21. The all-or-none law states that a muscle contraction either _____ or it _____ _____.

22. A constant state of partial contraction is called _____.

23. The muscle that is nonstriated and found in hollow structures is _____.

24. Smooth muscle contraction occurs without the regular rearrangement of _____.

25. Cardiac muscle is under the control of the _____ nervous system.

26. Fibrillation of cardiac muscle can result in _____.

27. Prime movers are _____.

28. _____ assist the prime movers.

29. Muscles found directly under the skin are _____ muscles.

30. _____ is muscle pain.

B. MATCHING

Match the term on the right with the definition on the left.

31. _____ striated muscle

32. _____ electrical cell membrane

33. _____ delicate connective tissue

34. _____ individual bundles of cells

35. _____ surrounds whole muscle

36. _____ dark bands of protein

37. _____ light of protein

38. _____ forms irregular curtain

39. _____ inside minus outside plus

40. _____ muscle impulse

41. _____ contain ATP molecule

42. _____ only in muscle tissue

43. _____ tension remains the same

44. _____ rapid uncontrolled contraction

45. _____ fixed attachment of muscle

46. _____ movable attachment of muscle

47. _____ prime mover

a. resting potential

b. phosphocreatine

c. trapezius

d. myosin

e. isotonic contraction

f. origin

g. fibrillation

h. insertion

i. skeletal

j. fascicle

k. action potential

l. sarcolemma

m. actin

n. zygomaticus

o. sarcoplasmic reticulum

p. myosin filaments

q. endomysium

48. _____ draw scalp backward   r. epimysium

49. _____ smiling muscle   s. agonists

50. _____ between the neck and clavicle   t. occipitalis

C. KEY TERMS

Use the text to look up the following terms. Write the definition or explanation.

51. Action potential: _____

_____

52. All-or-none law: _____

_____

53. Antagonists: _____

_____

54. Bands: _____

_____

55. Contracture: _____

_____

56. Cramps: _____

_____

57. Electrical potential: _____

_____

58. Fascicle: _____

_____

59. Fibrillation: _____

_____

60. H band: _____

_____

61. Hypertrophy: _____

_____

62. I band: _____

_____

63. Insertion: _____

_____

64. Isometric activity: _____

_____

65. Isotonic activity: _____

_____

66. Motor unit: _____

_____

67. Muscle twitch: _____

_____

68. Myalgia: _____

_____

69. Perimysium: _____

_____

70. Phosphocreatine: _____

_____

71. Psoas: _____

_____

72. Sarcotubular system: _____

_____

73. Synergists: _____

_____

74. T system: _____

_____

D. LABELING EXERCISE

75. Label the superficial muscles as indicated in Figure 9-1.

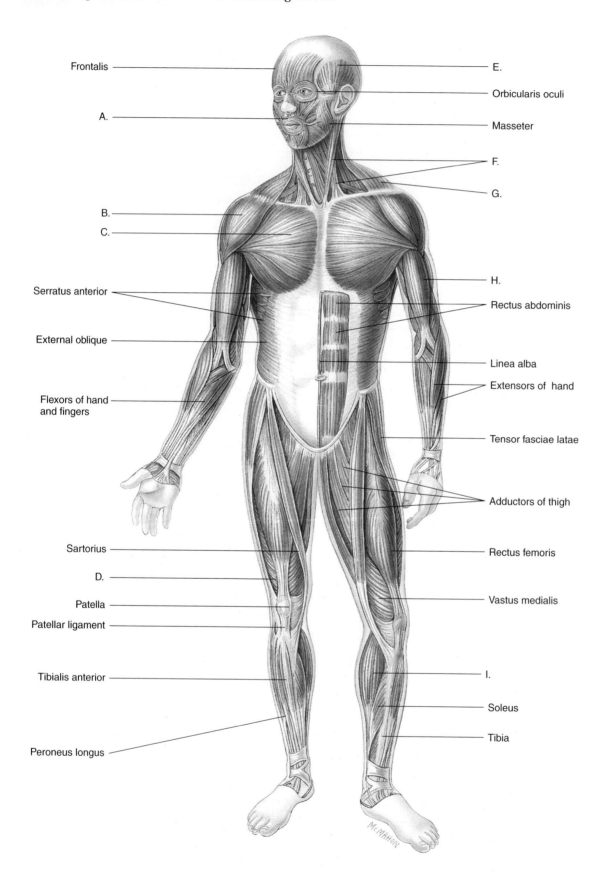

Frontalis

A.

Serratus anterior

External oblique

Flexors of hand and fingers

Sartorius

D.

Patella

Patellar ligament

Tibialis anterior

Peroneus longus

E.

Orbicularis oculi

Masseter

F.

G.

B.

C.

H.

Rectus abdominis

Linea alba

Extensors of hand

Tensor fasciae latae

Adductors of thigh

Rectus femoris

Vastus medialis

I.

Soleus

Tibia

a. _____

b. _____

c. _____

d. _____

e. _____

f. _____

g. _____

h. _____

i. _____

76. Label the superficial muscles as indicated in Figure 9-2.

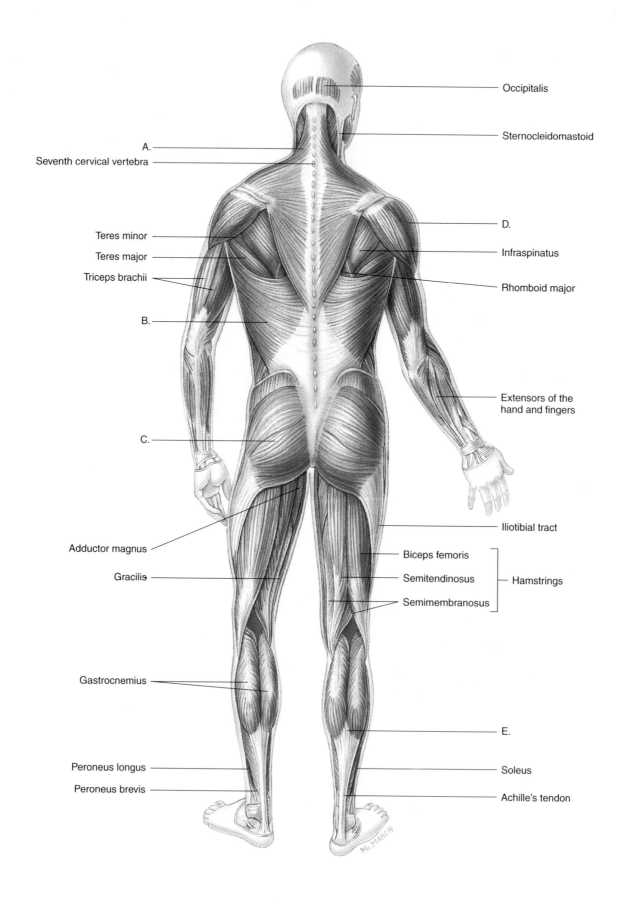

Occipitalis

Sternocleidomastoid

A.

Seventh cervical vertebra

D.

Teres minor

Infraspinatus

Teres major

Triceps brachii

Rhomboid major

B.

Extensors of the
hand and fingers

C.

Iliotibial tract

Adductor magnus

Biceps femoris

Gracilis

Semitendinosus

Hamstrings

Semimembranosus

Gastrocnemius

E.

Peroneus longus

Soleus

Peroneus brevis

Achille's tendon

a. _____
b. _____
c. _____
d. _____
e. _____

E. COLORING EXERCISE

77. Using Figure 9-3, color the gluteus maximus red, biceps femoris (long head) blue, biceps femoris (short head) yellow, soleus green and calcaneal tendon orange.

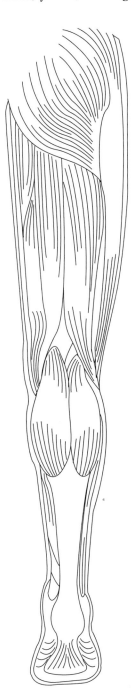

F. CRITICAL THINKING

Answer the following questions in complete sentences.

78. Why should weightlifters do aerobic exercises for maximal physical fitness?

79. Explain two ways in which prolonged exertion during hot weather might cause muscles to malfunction?

80. Why does stimulation of nerves with electrical current help stave off muscle atrophy for a short period of time?

81. Explain the function of troponin and tropomyosin and what negates them.

82. On what does the strength of contractions depend? Explain.

83. Identify age-related changes in the muscle system. Explain what a sports medicine physician and a massage therapist can do to help.

G. CROSSWORD PUZZLE

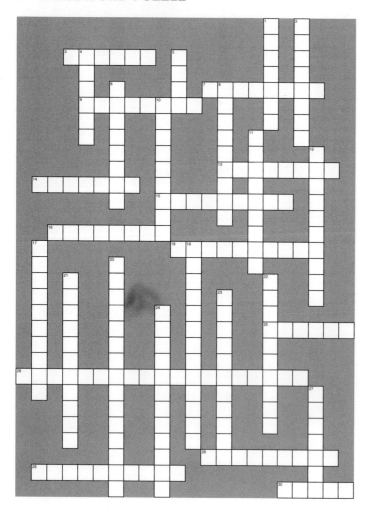

Complete the crossword puzzle using the following clues.

ACROSS

3. Muscle found in hollow body structures
7. Contraction when lifting a weight
9. Skeletal muscle type
13. Muscle that closes the jaw
14. Muscle pain
15. Movable muscle attachment
16. Muscle that protrudes the lower lip
18. Electrically polarized cell membrane
25. Fixed muscle attachment
26. Muscle that moves the head
28. Activity from tension against muscles
29. Muscle that compresses the cheek
30. Thin filaments of protein

DOWN

1. Injection site in the arm
2. Muscle inflammation
4. Thick protein filament in muscle cells
5. Constant state of partial contraction
6. Inhibitor substance
8. Area between Z lines
10. Muscle between the neck and clavicle
11. Skeletal muscle bundles
12. Muscle that raises the mandible
17. Muscles that assist the prime mover
19. Neurotransmitter substance
20. Rapid source of high-energy ATP
21. Increase in muscle size
22. Actin united with myosin
23. Smiling and laughing muscles
24. Rapid, uncontrolled contraction of heart cells
27. Prime mover

CHAPTER QUIZ

1. Muscles make up what percentage of body weight?

   a. 10–20%
   b. 20–30%
   c. 30–40%
   d. 40–50%
   e. 50–60%

2. The longest and most slender muscle fibers are the
   a. smooth
   b. skeletal
   c. cardiac
   d. none of the above

3. The entire muscle consists of a number of skeletal muscle bundles called
   a. perimysium
   b. myosin
   c. fasciculi
   d. actin
   e. none of the above

4. The sarcomere is the area between two
   a. Z bands
   b. H bands
   c. I bands
   d. A bands
   e. none of the above

5. The layer of areolar tissue covering the whole muscle trunk is called
   a. fascicle
   b. fasciculi
   c. epimysium
   d. fascia
   e. none of the above

6. The light bands are the
   a. A bands
   b. Z lines
   c. H bands
   d. I bands
   e. none of the above

7. The sarcotubular system is made up of the sarcoplasmic reticulum and the
   a. T system
   b. H system
   c. sarcomere
   d. vesicle system
   e. none of the above

8. On the average, a single motor nerve fiber innervates about how many muscle cells?
   a. 100
   b. 150
   c. 200
   d. 250
   e. none of the above

9. Which of the following properties do muscle cells NOT possess?
   a. excitability
   b. conductivity
   c. contractility
   d. elasticity
   e. none of the above

10. Which of the following is a neurotransmitter?
    a. acetylcholine
    b. myosin
    c. actin
    d. tropomyosin
    e. none of the above

11. Muscle contraction is
    a. resting potential
    b. electrical potential
    c. action potential
    d. none of the above

12. Calcium negates the effect of
    a. myosin
    b. troponin
    c. actin
    d. sodium
    e. none of the above

13. The sodium–potassium pump restores
    a. resting potential
    b. electrical potential
    c. action potential
    d. none of the above

14. Actin was discovered in
    a. 1868
    b. 1934
    c. 1942
    d. 1960
    e. none of the above

15. Which of the following retains the same width during contraction?
    a. A bands
    b. I bands
    c. H bands
    d. Z lines
    e. none of the above

16. Which of the following moves apart at the end of a contraction?
    a. A bands
    b. I bands
    c. H bands
    d. Z lines
    e. none of the above

17. ATP is synthesized by all of the following EXCEPT
    a. glycolysis
    b. Krebs' citric acid cycle
    c. electron transport
    d. breakdown of phosphocreatine
    e. none of the above

18. Which of the following is a rapid source of high-energy ATP for muscle contraction?
    a. glycolysis
    b. Krebs' citric acid cycle
    c. electron transport
    d. breakdown of phosphocreatine
    e. none of the above

19. Which of the following does a contraction NOT depend on?
    a. strength of stimulus
    b. duration of stimulus
    c. speed of stimulus
    d. temperature
    e. none of above

20. Muscle remains at constant length but tension increases. What type of contraction is this?
    a. isotonic
    b. isometric
    c. tonal
    d. none of above

21. Muscle shortens and thickens while tension remains constant. What type of contraction is this?
    a. isotonic
    b. isometric
    c. tonal
    d. none of above

22. Some muscles will always be contracting while others are at rest. What type of contraction is this?
    a. isotonic
    b. isometric
    c. tonal
    d. none of above

23. Two of the three kinds of muscle in the body are uninucleated; they are
    a. smooth and cardiac
    b. smooth and skeletal
    c. cardiac and skeletal
    d. none of above

24. Contraction is fastest in which kind of muscle?
    a. smooth
    b. cardiac
    c. skeletal
    d. none of above

25. The wide, flat attachment of muscle to bone is called
    a. ligament
    b. tendon
    c. insertion
    d. aponeurosis
    e. origin

26. The attachment of the biceps to the forearm is the
    a. agonist
    b. insertion
    c. origin
    d. ligament
    e. none of above

27. Muscles that straighten a joint are called
    a. agonists
    b. synergists
    c. insertions
    d. antagonists
    e. origins

28. An increase in muscle size is called
    a. atrophy
    b. myositis
    c. hypertrophy
    d. myalgia
    e. myasthenia gravis

29. Muscle weakness is called
    a. atrophy
    b. myositis
    c. hypertrophy
    d. myalgia
    e. myasthenia gravis

30. Inflammation of muscle tissue is called
    a. atrophy
    b. myositis
    c. hypertrophy
    d. myalgia
    e. myasthenia gravis

CHAPTER 10　THE NERVOUS SYSTEM: INTRODUCTION, SPINAL CORD AND SPINAL NERVES

CHAPTER OBJECTIVES

After studying this chapter, you should be able to:

1. Name the major subdivisions of the nervous system.
2. Classify the different types of neuroglia cells.
3. List the structural and functional classification of neurons.
4. Explain how a neuron transmits a nerve impulse.
5. Name the different types of neural tissues and their definitions.
6. Describe the structure of the spinal cord.
7. Name and number the spinal nerves.

ACTIVITIES

A. COMPLETION

Fill in the blank spaces with the correct term.

1. Being a _____ center and a _____ network is a function of the nervous system.

2. The control center for the entire system is the _____ _____ _____.

3. The sensory system, also named the _____ _____ _____, is a subdivision of the _____ _____ _____.

4. Motor neurons are part of the _____ _____ _____.

5. The speeding up of activity is a function of the _____ _____ portion of the ANS.

6. _____ slows down the system, whereas _____ speeds it up.

7. A nerve is a bundle of _____.

8. The nerve glue is the _____ cell.

9. _____ cells form myelin sheaths around nerve fibers.

10. The star-shaped _____ prevents toxic substances from entering the brain.

11. Protein synthesis occurs in the _____ _____, also called _____ _____.

12. The branches of trees on the nerve cell are the _____.

13. Peripheral axons are enclosed in fatty _____ sheaths.

14. Most neurons of the brain are _____.

15. Myelin gaps are called _____ _____.

16. The transmission of impulses is handled by the _____ neurons.

17. The efferent neurons are multipolar, the afferent neurons are _____.

18. The act of salivating would be caused by a _____ neuron.

19. The three types of ions involved in nerve impulses are _____, _____ and _____.

20. Reversal of electrical charge is _____.

21. When the outside of a nerve is positively charged and the inside is negatively charged, the condition is known as the _____ _____.

22. The nerve impulse is a self-propagating wave of _____.

23. The gap between the axon of one nerve and the dendrite of another is referred to as the _____.

24. The impulse is carried across the gap by _____.

25. An involuntary reaction to an external stimulus is called a _____.

26. The gray matter on the brain's surface is known as the _____.

27. The spider layer of the meninges is the _____ _____.

28. The sensory root of the spinal cord is the _____ _____.

29. There are _____ pairs of cervical nerves.

30. External stimuli affect _____ neurons.

B. MATCHING

Match the term on the right with the definition on the left.

31. _____ control center

32. _____ motor neuron

33. _____ sensory neurons

34. _____ majority of brain cells

35. _____ neurons with multiple dendrites

36. _____ neurolemmocytes

37. _____ myelin sheath gaps

38. _____ association neuron

39. _____ creates action potential

40. _____ gap between neurons

41. _____ epinephrine

42. _____ involuntary reaction

43. _____ like male hormones

44. _____ fiber bundle inside the CNS

45. _____ delicate mother

46. _____ spinal gray matter

a. reflex

b. adrenalin

c. pia mater

d. neurofibril nodes

e. synapse

f. cervical nerves

g. horn

h. anabolic steroids

i. CNS

j. efferent

k. internuncial

l. sensory

m. microglia

n. depolarization

o. neuroglia

p. tract

47. _____ dorsal root
48. _____ ventral root
49. _____ C1–C8
50. _____ phagocytosis of microbes

q. afferent
r. motor
s. Schwann cells
t. multipolar

C. KEY TERMS

Use the text to look up the following terms. Write the definition or explanation.

51. Acetylcholine: _____

_____

52. All-or-none law: _____

_____

53. Autonomic nervous system: _____

_____

54. Bipolar neurons: _____

_____

55. Chromatophilic substance or Nissl bodies: _____

_____

56. Cortex: _____

_____

57. Depolarization: _____

_____

58. Dopamine: _____

_____

59. Dura mater: _____

_____

60. Ependymal cells: _____

_____

61. Ganglia: _____

_____

62. Membrane or resting potential: _____

_____

63. Myelin sheath: _____

_____

64. Nerve: _____

_____

65. Nodes of Ranvier/neurofibril nodes: _____

_____

66. Oligodendroglia:_____

_____

67. Posterior or dorsal gray horn: _____

_____

68. Reflex: _____

_____

69. Repolarization: _____

_____

70. Schwann cells/neurolemmocytes: _____

_____

71. Serotonin: _____

_____

72. Somatic nervous system: _____

_____

73. Spinal meninges: _____

_____

74. Unipolar neurons: _____

_____

D. LABELING EXERCISE

75. Label the nerve cells as indicated in Figure 10-1.

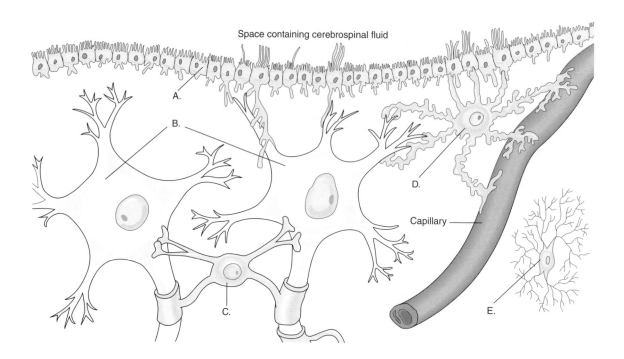

a. _____

b. _____

c. _____

d. _____

e. _____

76. Label the parts of the neuron as indicated in Figure 10-2.

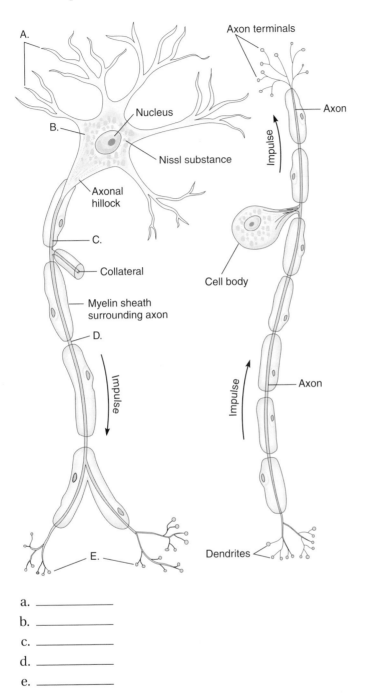

a. _____

b. _____

c. _____

d. _____

e. _____

E. COLORING EXERCISE

77. Using Figure 10-3, color the cervical spinal nerves red, the thoracic spinal nerves green, the lumbar spinal nerves yellow and the sacral spinal nerves blue.

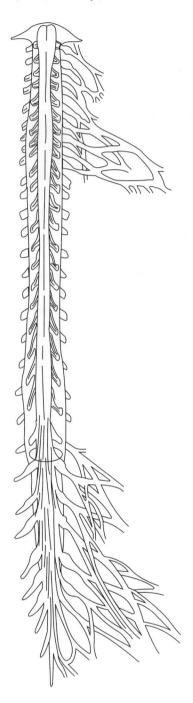

F. CRITICAL THINKING

Answer the following questions in complete sentences.

78. Explain how the sympathetic and parasympathetic systems work during a "fight or flight" experience.

79. Why is an efferent neuron multipolar?

80. Why do myelin covered neurons carry an action potential faster than an uncovered neuron?

81. Why doesn't acetylcholine remain on the postsynaptic neuron?

82. Using the five components of the reflex arc, explain the body's reaction to a hand on a hot surface.

83. How does the reflex action help maintain homeostasis?

G. CROSSWORD PUZZLE

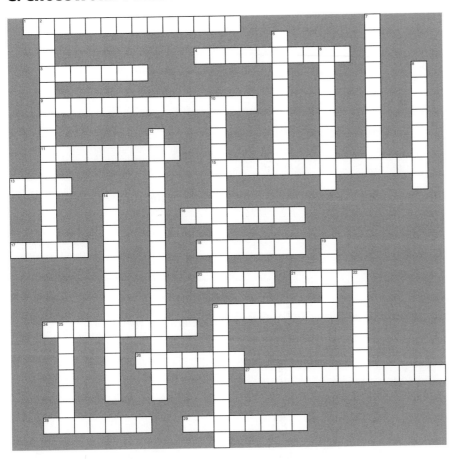

Complete the crossword puzzle using the following clues.

ACROSS

1. Sympathetic neurotransmitter

3. Nerve cell groups

4. Neurons that have several dendrites and one axon

9. Creates action potential

11. Receive stimuli

13. Long extension of a nerve cell body

15. Recharge nerves

16. Protective membrane

DOWN

2. Semirigid rows

5. Line brain ventricles

6. Spider layer

7. Downer

8. Motor neuron

10. Association neuron

12. Serotonin, endorphins

14. Parasympathetic neurotransmitter

19. Bundle of nerve cells

ACROSS	DOWN

ACROSS

17. Bundle inside the CNS

18. One axon, one dendrite

20. Cells that support and protect

21. Gray matter in spinal cord

23. Resting potential

24. Star shaped

26. Afferent neuron

27. Uppers

28. Nerve cells

29. Cells with only one process

DOWN

22. Kind of cells that form myelin sheaths

23. Do phagocytosis

25. Gap between neurons

CHAPTER QUIZ

1. The nervous system shares in the maintenance of homeostasis with which system?
   a. respiratory
   b. endocrine
   c. skeletal
   d. digestive
   e. muscular

2. The system that conducts impulses from the brain and spinal cord to skeletal muscles is the
   a. parasympathetic
   b. sympathetic
   c. autonomic
   d. somatic
   e. afferent

3. The "glue" cells that perform the function of support and protection are
   a. neurons
   b. astrocytes
   c. neuroglia
   d. ependymal
   e. Schwann

4. Oligodendroglia are found in the
   a. brain and spinal cord
   b. heart
   c. fingers
   d. muscles
   e. lungs

5. Phagocytosis is performed by
   a. astrocytes
   b. oligodendroglia
   c. microglia
   d. ependymal cells
   e. Schwann cells

6. The cells that make up the myelin sheath are
   a. astrocytes
   b. oligodendroglia
   c. microglia
   d. ependymal cells
   e. Schwann cells

7. The cells that line the cavities in brain and spinal cord are
   a. astrocytes
   b. oligodendroglia
   c. microglia
   d. ependymal cells
   e. Schwann cells

8. Nissl bodies are attached to
   a. mitochondria
   b. endoplasmic reticulum
   c. lysosome
   d. Golgi bodies
   e. neurofibrils

9. Neurolemmocytes are also known as
   a. astrocytes
   b. oligodendroglia
   c. microglia
   d. ependymal cells
   e. Schwann cells

10. A neuron with one axon and one dendrite is known as
    a. unipolar
    b. bipolar
    c. multipolar

11. Receptors are
    a. afferent neurons
    b. efferent neurons
    c. association neurons
    d. internuncial neurons

12. Reaction neurons are
    a. afferent neurons
    b. efferent neurons
    c. association neurons
    d. internuncial neurons

13. The sodium pump is used to maintain the
    a. action potential
    b. electrical potential
    c. membrane
    d. depolarization
    e. repolarization

14. Which of the following is NOT a neurotransmitter?
    a. acetylcholine
    b. norepinephrine
    c. serotonin
    d. dopamine
    e. none of above

15. The smallest, simplest pathway to receive and process a stimulus is the
    a. reflex
    b. CNS
    c. ANS
    d. neuroglia
    e. none of above

16. Some of the most commonly abused drugs are
    a. steroids
    b. depressants
    c. stimulants
    d. hallucinogens
    e. all of above

17. Ganglia are found
    a. in the brain
    b. in the cortex
    c. in a tract
    d. outside the brain
    e. none of above

18. Gray matter is found in the
    a. cortex
    b. myelin
    c. neuroglia
    d. nerve tracts
    e. none of above

19. The tough mother is the
    a. pia mater
    b. dura mater
    c. arachnoid mater

20. The layer containing numerous blood vessels and nerves is the
    a. pia mater
    b. dura mater
    c. arachnoid mater

21. The spider layer is the
    a. pia mater
    b. dura mater
    c. arachnoid matter

22. Serous fluid is found in the
    a. pia mater
    b. dura mater
    c. arachnoid mater
    d. subdural space

23. Spinal taps are done in which region of the spine?
    a. cervical
    b. thoracic
    c. lumbar
    d. sacral

24. Meninges are separated from the vertebrae by the
    a. subdural space
    b. epidural space
    c. subarachnoid space

25. The functions of the spinal cord include
    a. reflex/respiration
    b. reflex/emotion
    c. reflex/cogitation
    d. reflex/conveyance

CHAPTER 11   THE NERVOUS SYSTEM: THE BRAIN, CRANIAL NERVES, AUTONOMIC NERVOUS SYSTEM AND THE SPECIAL SENSES

CHAPTER OBJECTIVES

After studying this chapter, you should be able to:

1. List the principal parts of the brain.
2. Name the functions of the cerebrospinal fluid.
3. List the principal functions of the major parts of the brain.
4. List the 12 cranial nerves and their functions.
5. Name the parts of the autonomic nervous system and describe how it functions.
6. Describe the basic anatomy of the sense organs and explain how they function.

ACTIVITIES

A. COMPLETION

Fill in the blank spaces with the correct term.

1. The brain is protected by the _____ _____ and the _____.

2. The brain weighs _____ _____.

3. The three cranial meninges are the _____ mater, the _____ mater and the _____ mater.

4. The bridge of nerve fibers connecting the two sides of the brain is the _____ _____.

5. The third and fourth ventricles are connected by the _____ _____.

6. The area contained within the medulla having dispersed gray matter is the _____ _____.

7. The midbrain contains the _____ _____ _____.

8. The diencephalon is divided into the _____ and the _____.

9. The optic tracts and optic chiasma are within the _____.

10. The mammillary bodies are involved in _____ and _____ _____.

11. The superior part of the diencephalon that plays a role in conscious recognition of pain is the _____.

12. The surface of the cerebrum made up of gray matter is known as the _____ _____.

13. The right and left hemispheres of the brain are separated by the _____ _____.

14. The _____ lobe is behind the frontal lobe.

15. Deep within the lateral sulcus is the _____.

16. The second largest portion of the brain is the _____.

17. The autonomic nervous system, a subdivision of the peripheral nervous system, has two parts; they are the _____ and the _____.

18. There are _____ pairs of cranial nerves.

19. The sense of smell is the _____ sense.

20. In the cilia that detect odors are _____.

21. The _____ _____ actually function as the receptors of the taste cells.

22. There are four taste sensations; they are _____, _____, _____ and _____.

23. The black layer of the eye, which absorbs light, is the _____.

24. The portion of the eye that regulates the amount of light that enters the eye is the _____.

25. The area producing the sharpest vision is the _____ _____.

26. The two openings on the medial side of the middle ear are _____ _____ and the _____ _____.

27. The vestibule and the semicircular canals are involved in _____.

28. Inflammation of brain tissue is called _____.

29. _____ _____ is characterized by tremors of the hand.

30. Brain damage during brain development or the birth process can result in _____ _____.

B. MATCHING

Match the term on the right with the definition on the left.

31. _____ protect the brain

32. _____ cavities within the brain

33. _____ shock absorber for the CNS

34. _____ contains ascending and descending tracts

35. _____ bridge brain and spinal cord

36. _____ superior part of the diencephalon

37. _____ mesencephalon

38. _____ groove in the brain

39. _____ connects cerebral hemispheres

40. _____ deep in the lateral sulcus

41. _____ shaped like a butterfly

42. _____ fight or flight

43. _____ taste buds

44. _____ transparent front of the eye

45. _____ eye liquid

a. sulci

b. thalamus

c. papillae

d. otitis media

e. corpus callosum

f. cornea

g. stapes

h. aqueous humor

i. cerebrospinal fluid

j. pons varolii

k. eustachian tube

l. cerebellum

m. cranial meninges

n. malleus

o. medulla oblongata

46. _____ hammer

47. _____ stirrup

48. _____ tympanic membrane

49. _____ from the ear to the pharynx

50. _____ middle ear infection

p. sympathetic ANS

q. midbrain

r. insula

s. ventricles

t. eardrum

C. KEY TERMS

Use the text to look up the following terms. Write the definition or explanation.

51. Anesthesiologist: _____

_____

52. Auditory/eustachian tube: _____

_____

53. Auricle: _____

_____

54. Autonomic nervous system: _____

_____

55. Cerebral aqueduct/aqueduct of Sylvius: _____

_____

56. Cerebrum: _____

_____

57. Ciliary body: _____

_____

58. Conjunctivitis: _____

_____

59. Decussation pyramids: _____

_____

60. External auditory meatus: _____

_____

61. Fovea centralis: _____

_____

62. Infundibulum: _____

_____

63. Interventricular foramen/foramen of Monroe: _____

_____

64. Mammillary bodies: _____

_____

65. Occipital lobe: _____

_____

66. Optic chiasma: _____

_____

67. Optic disk: _____

_____

68. Oval window: _____

_____

69. Parasympathetic division: _____

_____

70. Parkinson's disease: _____

_____

71. Pons varolii: _____

_____

72. Reticular formation: _____

_____

73. Retina: _____

_____

74. Rhodopsin: _____

_____

75. Round window: _____

_____

76. Sulci: _____

_____

77. Taste cells: _____

_____

78. Ventral cerebral peduncles: _____

_____

79. Ventricles: _____

_____

80. Vitreous humor: _____

_____

D. LABELING EXERCISE

81. Label the parts of the ear as indicated in Figure 11-1.

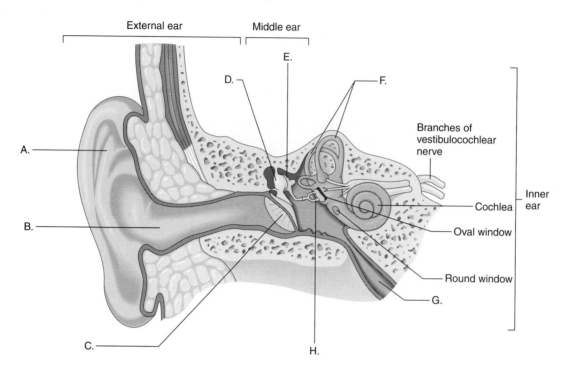

a. _____

b. _____

c. _____

d. _____

e. _____

f. _____

g. _____

h. _____

82. Label the parts of the eye as indicated in Figure 11-2.

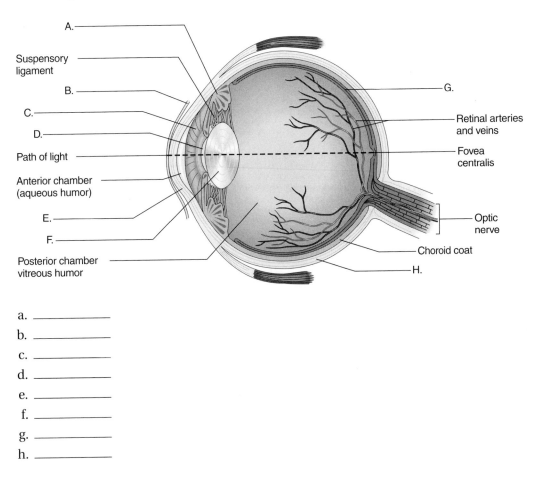

a. _____

b. _____

c. _____

d. _____

e. _____

f. _____

g. _____

h. _____

E. COLORING EXERCISE

83. Using Figure 11-3, color the cerebrum red, the occipital lobe green, the cerebellum blue, the midbrain orange, the pons yellow and the medulla brown.

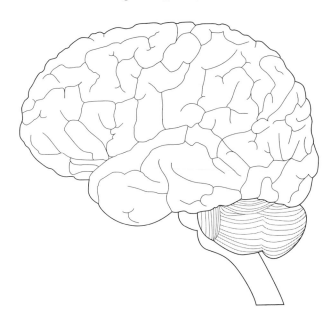

F. CRITICAL THINKING

Answer the following questions in complete sentences.

84. Explain the mechanism of the fight or flight response.

85. What is the importance of the hypothalamus?

86. How would damage to the cerebellum affect the body?

87. How can the common cold affect the sense of taste?

88. How does flying in an airplane affect hearing?

89. Why should children not go to school when they have "pinkeye"?

90. Why do some middle-aged people have to get reading glasses?

91. What would be a possible treatment for glaucoma?

92. Identify age-related changes in the nervous system. Briefly explain the effects these changes have on older adults.

93. Of the career options associated with the nervous system, select the one that is most interesting to you. Tell why you consider this option as a potential career.

94. Distinguish between a psychiatrist and a psychologist.

G. CROSSWORD PUZZLE

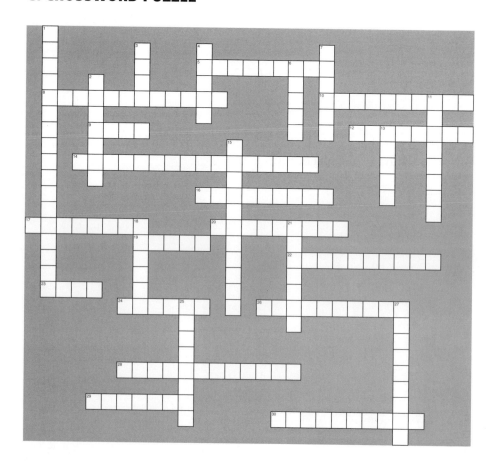

Complete the crossword puzzle using the following clues.

ACROSS

5. Nerve that controls head movements

8. Diencephalon part attached to the pituitary

9. Eyeball's colored part

10. Decrease in near vision

12. Seizures

14. Nerve that senses taste

16. Smallest of the cranial nerves

17. Relays sensory impulses

19. Retina cells that produce color

20. Nerve that controls smell

22. Largest of the cranial nerves

23. Retina cells very sensitive to light

24. Nerve that controls tear glands

26. Nerve that controls eyelid movement

28. Surrounds the third ventricle

29. Earwax

30. Headache

DOWN

1. Nerve that controls balance and hearing

2. Outer part of the ear

3. Brain foids

4. Nerve that conveys sensation in the larynx

6. Nerve that conveys vision impulses

7. Nearsightedness

11. Elevations of the tongue

13. Anvil

15. Nerve that controls swallowing

18. Eye's outermost layer

21. Lockjaw

25. Nerve that controls eyeball movement

27. Rod pigment

CHAPTER QUIZ

1. The disease that produces convulsive seizures is
   a. epilepsy
   b. cerebral palsy
   c. otitis media
   d. tetanus
   e. encephalitis

2. The disease that produces infection in the middle ear is
   a. epilepsy
   b. cerebral palsy
   c. otitis media
   d. tetanus
   e. encephalitis

3. The disease that produces defective muscular coordination is
   a. epilepsy
   b. cerebral palsy
   c. otitis media
   d. tetanus
   e. encephalitis

4. Farsightedness is
   a. myopia
   b. hyperopia
   c. presbyopia
   d. glaucoma

5. An accommodation disease of aging is
   a. myopia
   b. hyperopia
   c. presbyopia
   d. glaucoma

6. A disease that causes destruction of the retina is
   a. myopia
   b. hyperopia
   c. presbyopia
   d. glaucoma

7. Nearsightedness is
   a. myopia
   b. hyperopia
   c. presbyopia
   d. glaucoma

8. The part of the ear allowing for pressure equalization is the
   a. stapes
   b. vestibule
   c. auricle
   d. tympanum
   e. eustachian tube

9. The part of the ear allowing for balance is the
   a. stapes
   b. vestibule
   c. auricle
   d. tympanum
   e. eustachian tube

10. The part of the ear acting like a drum head is the
    a. stapes
    b. vestibule
    c. auricle
    d. tympanic membrane
    e. eustachian tube

11. Night blindness can be caused by a deficiency of
    a. vitamin A
    b. vitamin D
    c. vitamin K
    d. vitamin B
    e. vitamin E

12. The ability to see color is due to
    a. rods
    b. choroid
    c. cones
    d. sclera
    e. lens

13. The white, outermost layer of the eye is the
    a. pupil
    b. choroid
    c. retina
    d. sclera
    e. lens

14. The cells of the retina are
    a. unipolar
    b. bipolar
    c. multipolar

15. Glaucoma is caused by a defect of the
    a. sclera
    b. vitreous humor
    c. aqueous humor
    d. lens
    e. choroid

16. Rhodopsin is found in the
    a. rods
    b. sclera
    c. cones
    d. choroid
    e. lens

17. The actual taste function is found on the
    a. taste buds
    b. taste cells
    c. taste
    d. taste hairs

18. Chemoreceptors are used in the sense of
    a. taste
    b. sight
    c. smell
    d. hearing
    e. touch

19. The cranial nerves number
    a. 6
    b. 12
    c. 24
    d. 36
    e. 48

20. The neurotransmitter associated with the parasympathetic system is
    a. epinephrine
    b. adrenalin
    c. norepinephrine
    d. serotonin
    e. acetylcholine

21. Which of the following is NOT a function of the cerebellum?
    a. reflex
    b. coordination
    c. posture
    d. balance
    e. none of the above

22. Which lobe of the cerebrum evaluates hearing input?
    a. parietal
    b. frontal
    c. temporal
    d. occipital
    e. none of the above

23. Which lobe of the cerebrum is involved in visual input?
    a. parietal
    b. frontal
    c. temporal
    d. occipital
    e. none of the above

24. Which lobe of the cerebrum is involved in evaluating sensory information?
    a. parietal
    b. frontal
    c. temporal
    d. occipital
    e. none of the above

25. Which lobe of the cerebrum controls moods, aggression and motivation?
    a. parietal
    b. frontal
    c. temporal
    d. occipital
    e. none of the above

26. Each hemisphere has folds called
    a. gyri
    b. sulci
    c. fissures
    d. lobes
    e. none of the above

27. The mind controlling the body phenomenon is located in the
    a. thalamus
    b. hypothalamus
    c. midbrain
    d. cerebellum
    e. none of the above

28. The ventral cerebral peduncles are contained in the
    a. cerebellum
    b. cerebrum
    c. medulla oblongata
    d. midbrain
    e. none of the above

29. The foramen of Monroe connects
    a. sulci
    b. gyri
    c. ventricles
    d. lobes
    e. none of the above

30. Which of the following is NOT an area of the brainstem?
    a. medulla oblongata
    b. pons varolii
    c. midbrain
    d. none of the above

CHAPTER 12   THE ENDOCRINE SYSTEM

CHAPTER OBJECTIVES

After studying this chapter, you should be able to:

1. List the functions of hormones.
2. Classify hormones into their major chemical categories.
3. Describe how the hypothalamus of the brain controls the endocrine system.
4. Name the endocrine glands and state where they are located.
5. List the major hormones and their effects on the body.

ACTIVITIES

A. COMPLETION

Fill in the blank spaces with the correct term.

1. The hypothalamus sends directions to the pituitary gland by
   _____ _____.

2. Endocrine glands are ductless glands. This means they secrete their hormones directly
   into the _____.

3. Negative feedback means that when a hormone reaches a certain level, the gland's
   secretion is _____.

4. Hormones can be classified into _____ categories.

5. The simplest group of hormones are the modified _____ _____.

6. The second category of hormones are the _____ hormones.

7. _____ are the third kind of hormones.

8. Steroid hormones are soluble in _____.

9. Because they cannot diffuse across the intestinal lining, protein and modified amino
   acid hormones like insulin must be _____.

10. Anabolic steroids are variants of _____.

11. Athletes use anabolic steroids to build _____ _____.

12. The chemical signals of the hypothalamus are called _____ _____
    and _____-_____ _____.

13. The pituitary gland is also called the _____.

14. The pituitary gland has two lobes, the _____ and the _____ lobes.

15. The larger of the lobes produces _____ hormones.

16. TSH stimulates the _____ gland to produce its hormone.

17. MSH increases the production of melanin and this _____ the skin.

18. Luteinizing hormone stimulates _____ in the female.

19. ADH inhibits the body from excreting _____.

20. Oxytocin stimulates contraction of the uterus and also stimulates _____.

21. A goiter is an enlarged _____ gland.

22. To properly function, the thyroid gland must have _____.

23. The parathyroid glands consist of _____ cells and _____ cells.

24. The hormone from the parathyroid glands functions to balance _____ levels in the body.

25. The adrenal medulla secretes _____; the adrenal cortex secretes a number of hormones, the most important of which is _____.

26. The middle layer of the adrenal cortex secretes _____, which is also known as _____.

27. The sex hormones secreted by the inner layer of the adrenal cortex are _____.

28. The islets of Langerhans are located on the _____, and they produce the hormones _____ and _____.

29. Glycosuria is a condition of elevated sugar in the _____.

30. The thymus gland is important in the development of _____.

B. MATCHING

Match the term on the right with the definition on the left.

31. _____ secretes into blood

32. _____ have ducts

33. _____ simplest hormones

34. _____ stimulates or inhibits hormone release

35. _____ controls many glands

36. _____ stimulates cell metabolism

37. _____ darkens the skin

38. _____ maintains progesterone during pregnancy

39. _____ maintains water balance

40. _____ ADH deficiency

41. _____ stimulates lactation

42. _____ enlarged thyroid

43. _____ contains four iodine atoms

44. _____ hyperthyroidism

45. _____ lowers calcium level

46. _____ inhibits osteoblasts

47. _____ increases calcium absorption

48. _____ atop kidneys

49. _____ glucocorticoid hormone

50. _____ regulates blood glucose

a. adrenals

b. thyroxine

c. pituitary gland

d. cortisol

e. oxytocin

f. parathormone

g. prolactin

h. Graves' disease

i. vitamin D

j. MSH

k. modified amino acids

l. glucagon

m. calcitonin

n. diabetes insipidus

o. exocrine

p. vasopressin

q. neurosecretion

r. goiter

s. growth hormone

t. ductless glands

C. KEY TERMS

Use the text to look up the following terms. Write the definition or explanation.

51. Acidosis: _____

_____

52. Addison's disease: _____

_____

53. Adrenal glands/suprarenal glands: _____

_____

54. Adrenocorticotropic hormone/ACTH: _____

_____

55. Alpha cells:_____

_____

56. Androgens:_____

_____

57. Antidiuretic hormone/ADH/vasopressin:_____

_____

58. Beta cells: _____

_____

59. Chief cells: _____

_____

60. Cretinism: _____

_____

61. Cushing's syndrome: _____

_____

62. Estrogen: _____

_____

63. Exophthalmia:_____

_____

64. Graves' disease:_____

_____

65. Homeostasis:_____

_____

66. Hyperglycemia:_____

_____

67. Hypophysis: _____

_____

68. Melatonin: _____

_____

69. Myxedema: _____

_____

70. Negative feedback system: _____

_____

71. Oxyphil cells: _____

_____

72. Pineal gland/body: _____

_____

73. Polydipsia: _____

_____

74. Polyphagia: _____

_____

75. Polyuria: _____

_____

76. Releasing hormones: _____

_____

77. Releasing-inhibitory hormones: _____

_____

78. Thymosin: _____

_____

79. Thyroxine or tetraiodothyronine (T_4): _____

_____

80. Triiodothyronine (T_3): _____

_____

D. LABELING EXERCISE

81. Label the parathyroid glands and their cellular components as indicated in Figure 12-1.

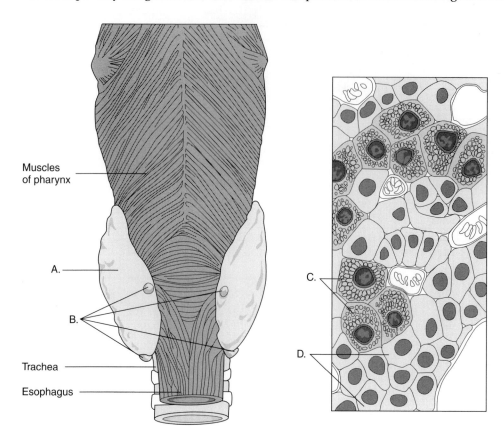

Muscles
of pharynx

A.

B.

Trachea

Esophagus

C.

D.

a. _____

b. _____

c. _____

d. _____

82. Label the endocrine glands as indicated in Figure 12-2.

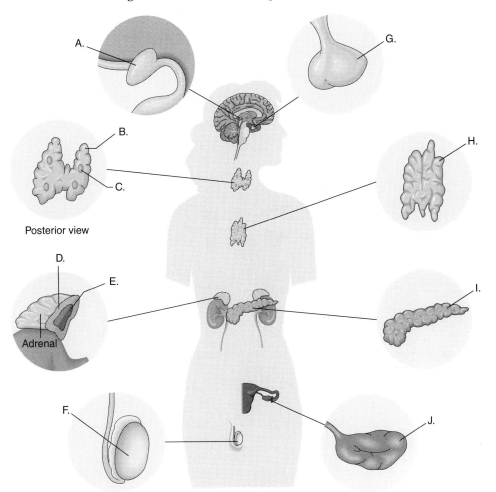

A.

G.

B.

H.

C.

Posterior view

D.

E.

Adrenal

I.

F.

J.

a. _____

b. _____

c. _____

d. _____

e. _____

f. _____

g. _____

h. _____

i. _____

j. _____

E. COLORING EXERCISE

83. Using Figure 12-3, color the corpus callosum red, the thalamus blue, the pineal gland green, the pituitary gland yellow and the hypothalamus brown.

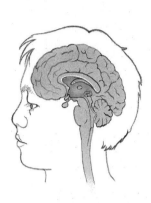
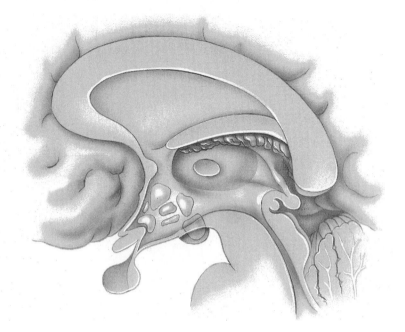

F. CRITICAL THINKING

Answer the following questions in complete sentences.

84. Why must hormones like insulin and oxytocin be injected?

85. Explain some of the dangers associated with overuse of anabolic steroids.

86. Why does excess secretion of growth hormone in childhood produce gigantism and in adulthood acromegaly?

87. Why are goiters much less common today than 100 years ago?

88. Explain the difference between the effects of hypothyroidism in adults and in children.

89. Explain the effects of hypoparathyroidism.

90. Differentiate between diabetes mellitus I and II.

91. Identify age-related changes to the endocrine system and one effective strategy for offsetting these changes.

92. Evaluate your interest and abilities for one of these career paths: nuclear medicine technologist, endocrinologist or diabetes dietician.

G. CROSSWORD PUZZLE

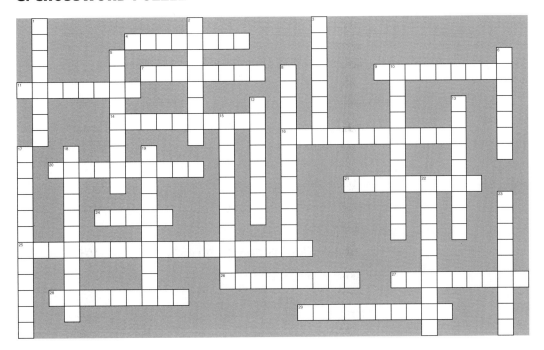

Complete the crossword puzzle using the following clues.

ACROSS

4. Stimulates uterine contraction
7. Hormone producing T lymphocytes
9. Pineal gland hormone
11. Secreted from the adrenal cortex
14. Enlarged hands and feet
16. Male sex hormone
20. Secreted by the thyroid gland
21. Adrenal sex hormones
24. Route for hormone transport
25. Bones become soft
26. Ductless glands
27. Stimulated by luteinizing hormone
28. Master gland of endocrine system
29. Pituitary gland

DOWN

1. Female sex hormone
2. Control the body's internal environment
3. Low blood pH
5. Stimulates milk production
6. Secreted by pancreatic islets
8. Inferior diencephalon
10. Fight or flight hormone
12. Adult hypothyroidism condition
13. Children's hypothyroidism
15. Regulates sodium reabsorption
17. Bulging eyes
18. Antidiuretic hormone
19. Intense food craving
22. Excess sugar in urine
23. Acts as vasoconstrictor

CHAPTER QUIZ

1. The gland crucial to the immune system is the
   a. pituitary
   b. thymus
   c. thyroid
   d. adrenal
   e. pineal

2. The gland responsible for the secretion of melatonin is the
   a. pituitary
   b. thymus
   c. thyroid
   d. adrenal
   e. pineal

3. The gland that secretes cortisol is the
   a. pituitary
   b. thymus
   c. thyroid
   d. adrenal
   e. pineal

4. The secretion that regulates the blood sugar level is
   a. cortisol
   b. thyroxin
   c. glucagon
   d. melatonin
   e. none of the above

5. A low blood sugar level can cause
   a. acidosis
   b. pancreatitis
   c. hypothyroidism
   d. goiter
   e. none of the above

6. Epinephrine is secreted by the
   a. pituitary
   b. thyroid
   c. thymus
   d. pancreas
   e. none of the above

7. Vitamin D increases the absorption of
   a. sodium
   b. calcium
   c. chlorine
   d. potassium
   e. none of the above

8. Which of the following glands needs iodine to function correctly?
   a. thymus
   b. pituitary
   c. thyroid
   d. adrenal
   e. none of the above

9. ADH helps maintain proper water balance in the body. It is also called
   a. vasopressin
   b. adrenalin
   c. thymosin
   d. oxytocin
   e. none of the above

10. The hormone that stimulates ovary follicle development and sperm cell production is
    a. FSH
    b. MSH
    c. LH
    d. TSH
    e. none of the above

11. The master gland is controlled by the
    a. pituitary
    b. thalamus
    c. hypothalamus
    d. cerebellum
    e. none of the above

12. The hormones that can diffuse across cell membranes are the
    a. proteins
    b. steroids
    c. amino acids
    d. oxytocin
    e. none of the above

13. Which of the following is NOT a function of hormones?
    a. growth
    b. reproduction
    c. behavior patterns
    d. maturation
    e. none of the above

14. Which of the following organs controls water levels and electrolyte balance?
    a. pancreas
    b. liver
    c. kidneys
    d. heart
    e. none of the above

15. The production of T lymphocytes is done in the
    a. thyroid
    b. pituitary
    c. parathyroid
    d. thymus
    e. none of the above

16. Glycogen is stored for use between meals. It is stored in which organ?
    a. pancreas
    b. liver
    c. kidneys
    d. heart
    e. none of the above

17. The functions of the reproductive system are inhibited by
    a. thymosin
    b. melatonin
    c. renin
    d. thyroxine
    e. none of the above

18. The pineal gland secretes which two substances?
    a. melatonin/serotonin
    b. thyroxine/thymosin
    c. estrogen/progesterone
    d. ADH/oxytocin
    e. none of the above

19. Polyuria, polydipsia and polyphagia are associated with
    a. gigantism
    b. cretinism
    c. acromegaly
    d. diabetes
    e. none of the above

20. If blood glucose decreases excessively, fatty acids and what are released to cause acidosis?
    a. proteins
    b. sugar
    c. ketones
    d. steroids
    e. none of the above

21. Pancreatic juice is produced by
    a. acini cells
    b. alpha cells
    c. beta cells
    d. red cells
    e. none of the above

22. Insulin is produced by
    a. acini cells
    b. alpha cells
    c. beta cells
    d. red cells
    e. none of the above

23. Glucagon is produced by the
    a. acini cells
    b. alpha cells
    c. beta cells
    d. red cells
    e. none of the above

24. Androgens are produced by the
    a. acini cells
    b. alpha cells
    c. beta cells
    d. red cells
    e. none of the above

25. Overproduction of hormones by the adrenal cortex can lead to
    a. Addison's disease
    b. Graves' disease
    c. Cushing's syndrome
    d. cretinism
    e. none of the above

26. A bronzing of the skin is a symptom of which disease?
    a. Addison's disease
    b. Graves' disease
    c. Cushing's syndrome
    d. cretinism
    e. none of the above

27. The gland sitting atop the kidney is the
    a. pituitary
    b. adrenal
    c. thymus
    d. thyroid
    e. none of the above

28. Which of the following hormones is NOT secreted by the thyroid gland?
    a. tetraiodothyronine
    b. triiodothyronine
    c. calcitonin
    d. serotonin
    e. none of the above

29. Which of the following is NOT a disease of the thyroid gland?
    a. myxedema
    b. goiter
    c. Graves' disease
    d. cretinism
    e. none of the above

30. Which of the following stimulates milk production?
    a. FSH
    b. LTH
    c. MSH
    d. LH
    e. none of the above

CHAPTER 13   THE BLOOD

CHAPTER OBJECTIVES

After studying this chapter, you should be able to:

1. Describe the functions of blood.
2. Classify the different types of blood cells.
3. Describe the anatomy of erythrocytes relative to their function.
4. Compare the functions of the different leukocytes.
5. Explain how and where blood cells are formed.
6. Explain the clotting mechanism.
7. Name the different blood groups.

ACTIVITIES

A. COMPLETION

Fill in the blank spaces with the correct term.

1. Platelets are also called _____.

2. The white cells are the _____ and the red cells are the _____.

3. Blood transports oxygen from the lungs and _____ _____ to the lungs.

4. The regulation of water by the blood plays a role in the process of _____.

5. Neutrophils, eosinophils and basophils are the _____ leukocytes.

6. Of the three proteins in plasma, _____ is the one that plays a role in maintaining water balance.

7. _____ carries hormones to target organs.

8. Blood cell formation occurs in _____ _____.

9. Lymphocytes and monocytes are produced in certain _____ tissue.

10. Undifferentiated mesenchymal cells are called _____.

11. Some stem cells will become _____, and these mature into erythrocytes.

12. Red blood cells do not have a _____.

13. Heme contains the element _____.

14. Although leukocytes have a nucleus, they do not have any _____.

15. Leukocytes clean up foreign bodies by _____.

16. The destruction of certain bacteria is accomplished by the enzyme _____.

17. After they leave the blood and enter tissues, _____ increase in size.

18. Disk-shaped cellular fragments with a nucleus are the _____.

19. In the first stage of clotting, _____ is released.

20. In the second stage of clotting, prothrombin is converted to _____.

21. The formation of the clot is a result of the production of _____.

22. After the clot forms, the plasma remaining is called _____.

23. After tissue repair, fibrinolysis occurs; this is a _____ of the blood clot.

24. Clotting in an unbroken vessel is called _____.

25. A piece of a thrombus that breaks off is an _____.

26. Antigens on the red blood cell membrane are the basis of blood _____.

27. The universal donor is a person with blood type _____.

28. A genetically inherited blood clotting disease is _____.

29. Another hereditary blood disease causing suppressed hemoglobin production is _____.

30. Infectious mononucleosis is caused by the _____-_____ virus.

B. MATCHING

Match the term on the right with the definition on the left.

31. _____ erythrocyte
32. _____ thrombocyte
33. _____ 55% of blood
34. _____ granular leukocyte
35. _____ maintain osmotic pressure
36. _____ vital role in clotting
37. _____ stem cell
38. _____ red pigment
39. _____ no nuclei, no pigment
40. _____ enzyme that destroys certain bacteria
41. _____ involved in production of antibodies
42. _____ production of prothrombin activation
43. _____ clot retraction
44. _____ dissolution of clot
45. _____ piece of blood clot
46. _____ clumping red blood cells
47. _____ red cells destroyed
48. _____ suppressed hemoglobin production
49. _____ blood poisoning
50. _____ produce serotonin

a. leukocytes
b. septicemia
c. syneresis
d. hemolytic anemia
e. embolus
f. plasma
g. basophils
h. platelets
i. fibrinolysis
j. hematocytoblasts
k. fibrinogen
l. lymphocytes
m. thalassemia
n. albumin
o. red cell
p. thromboplastin
q. hemoglobin
r. lysozyme
s. agglutination
t. eosinophils

C. KEY TERMS

Use the text to look up the following terms. Write the definition or explanation.

51. Agglutination: _____

_____

52. Embolism: _____

_____

53. Erythrocytes: _____

_____

54. Fibrinogen: _____

_____

55. Globin: _____

_____

56. Globulins: _____

_____

57. Hematopoiesis: _____

_____

58. Hemophilia: _____

_____

59. Infarction: _____

_____

60. Macrophages: _____

_____

61. Megakaryocytes: _____

_____

62. Monocytes: _____

_____

63. Myeloid tissue/red bone marrow: _____

_____

64. Neutrophils: _____

_____

65. Plaque: _____

_____

66. Prothrombin: _____

_____

67. Rh blood group: _____

_____

68. Thrombin: _____

_____

69. Thromboplastin: _____

_____

70. Thrombus: _____

_____

D. LABELING EXERCISE

71. Label the blood cells as indicated in Figure 13-1.

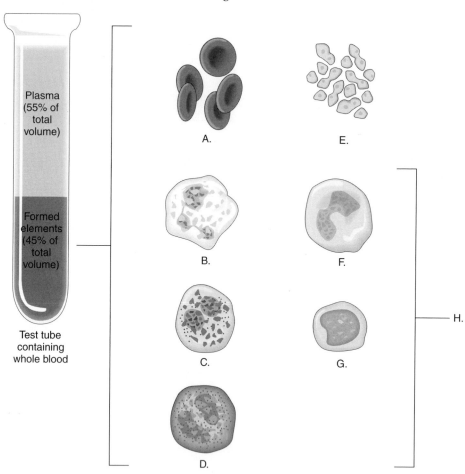

a. _____

b. _____

c. _____

d. _____

e. _____

f. _____

g. _____

h. _____

72. Label the various leukocytes as indicated in Figure 13-2.

White blood cells (leukocytes)

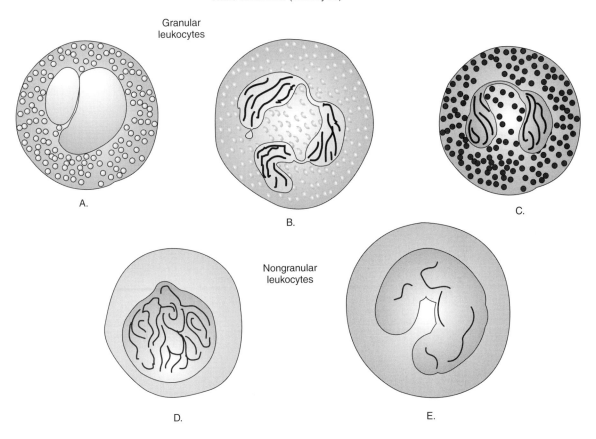

Granular
leukocytes

A.

B.

C.

Nongranular
leukocytes

D.

E.

a. _____
b. _____
c. _____
d. _____
e. _____

E. COLORING EXERCISE

73. Using Figure 13-3, color the prothrombin yellow, the thromboplastin blue, the thrombin green and the red cells red.

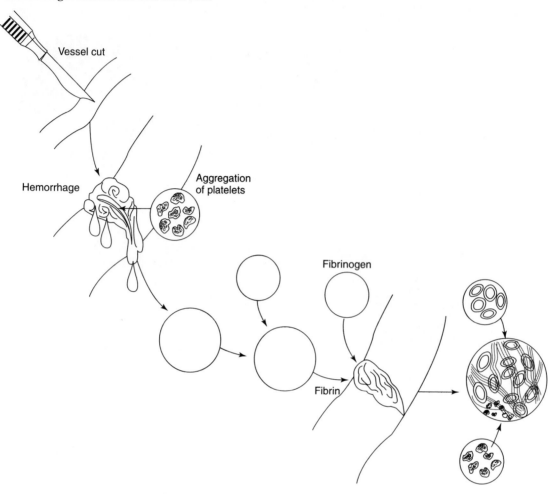

F. CRITICAL THINKING

Answer the following questions in complete sentences.

74. How does blood help regulate body water content?

75. Explain hematopoiesis.

76. Describe the primary function of erythrocytes.

77. Explain the clotting mechanism process.

78. Explain blood typing.

79. How is erythroblastosis fetalis developed?

80. How does sickle cell anemia work?

81. How can a clot cause death?

82. Explain the connection between the blood and vitamin K.

83. Explain why smoking may cause mental impairment.

84. Distinguish between a hematologist and an infectious disease specialist.

G. CROSSWORD PUZZLE

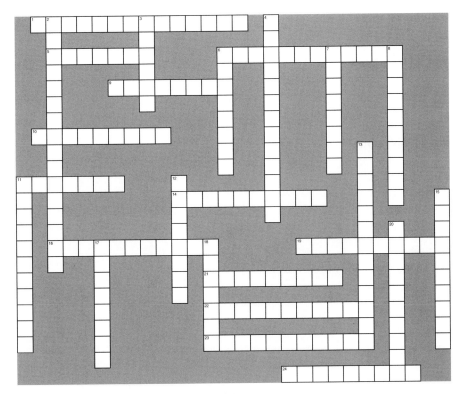

Complete the crossword puzzle using the following clues.

ACROSS

1. Prothrombin activator
5. *Anopheles* mosquito
6. Eating cells
9. Blood cancer
10. Clot retraction
11. Piece of blood clot
14. Red pigment
16. Suppressed hemoglobin production
19. Clotting disorder
21. Release heparin
22. Largest leukocytes
23. Most common leukocytes
24. Antibodies

DOWN

2. Stem cells
3. Cholesterol-containing mass
4. Red cells clump
6. Blood cells involved in clotting
7. Catalyst for fibrin
8. Blood poisoning
11. Combat irritants
12. Clot
13. Blood cell formation
15. Tissue killed
17. Bacteria destroyed in enzyme
18. Maintain osmotic pressure
20. Clotting

CHAPTER QUIZ

1. The fluid part of the blood is called
   a. erythrocytes
   b. leukocytes
   c. thrombocytes
   d. plasma
   e. none of the above

2. The amount of blood in the body is about
   a. 3–4 liters
   b. 6–7 liters
   c. 5–6 liters
   d. 4–5 liters
   e. none of the above

3. Which of the following is NOT transported by the blood?
   a. water
   b. lymph
   c. oxygen
   d. carbon dioxide
   e. none of the above

4. Which of the following parts of the blood play a role in temperature regulation?
   a. erythrocytes
   b. leukocytes
   c. water
   d. thrombocytes
   e. none of the above

5. Which of the following is NOT a granular leukocyte?
   a. lymphocyte
   b. neutrophil
   c. eosinophil
   d. basophil
   e. none of the above

6. The solid element of the blood responsible for clotting is the
   a. erythrocyte
   b. leukocyte
   c. thrombocyte
   d. albumin
   e. none of the above

7. Which of the following is NOT present in the plasma?
   a. water
   b. fibrinogen
   c. albumin
   d. globulin
   e. none of the above

8. Blood cells develop from all of the following EXCEPT
   a. mesenchymal cells
   b. stem cells
   c. hematocytoblasts
   d. lymphocytes
   e. none of the above

9. Proerythroblasts eventually become
   a. erythrocytes
   b. leukocytes
   c. thrombocytes
   d. lymphoblasts
   e. none of the above

10. Hemoglobin contains which of the following elements?
    a. sodium
    b. iron
    c. copper
    d. potassium
    e. none of the above

11. The number of red blood cells in the female's body is
    a. 5.4 million
    b. 2.6 million
    c. 5–9 thousand
    d. 4–5 hundred thousand
    e. none of the above

12. Neutrophils are the most common
    a. erythrocytes
    b. leukocytes
    c. thrombocytes
    d. lymphocytes
    e. none of the above

13. Which of the following are phagocytic?
    a. neutrophils
    b. eosinophils
    c. basophils
    d. platelets
    e. none of the above

14. Which of the following produce antihistamines?
    a. neutrophils
    b. eosinophils
    c. basophils
    d. platelets
    e. none of the above

15. Which of the following produce heparin?
    a. neutrophils
    b. eosinophils
    c. basophils
    d. platelets
    e. none of the above

16. Thrombocytes are produced in the red bone marrow from
    a. lymphocytes
    b. monocytes
    c. megakaryocytes
    d. macrophages
    e. none of the above

17. Prothrombin is produced in which stage of coagulation?
    a. first
    b. second
    c. third
    d. fourth
    e. none of the above

18. Fibrinogen is produced in which stage of coagulation?
    a. first
    b. second
    c. third
    d. fourth
    e. none of the above

19. The material that actually forms the clot is
    a. prothrombin
    b. fibrinogen
    c. thrombin
    d. fibrin
    e. none of the above

20. Clot retraction is called
    a. syneresis
    b. fibrinolysis
    c. hematopoiesis
    d. agglutination
    e. none of the above

21. Clot dissolution is called
    a. syneresis
    b. fibrinolysis
    c. hematopoiesis
    d. agglutination
    e. none of the above

22. Blood clumping is called
    a. syneresis
    b. fibrinolysis
    c. hematopoiesis
    d. agglutination
    e. none of the above

23. A blood clot in the brain blocking a vessel is called a(n)
    a. coronary thrombosis
    b. cerebral thrombosis
    c. embolus
    d. pulmonary embolism
    e. none of the above

24. Of the four blood groups, which of the following is the universal donor type?
    a. A
    b. B
    c. AB
    d. O
    e. none of the above

25. Of the four blood groups, which of the following is the universal recipient type?
    a. A
    b. B
    c. AB
    d. O
    e. none of the above

26. The hemolytic disease of the newborn is
    a. erythroblastosis fetalis
    b. hemophilia
    c. leukemia
    d. anemia
    e. none of the above

27. The anemia caused by the abnormal shape of red blood cells is
    a. hemolytic
    b. leukemia
    c. thalassemia
    d. hemophilia
    e. none of the above

28. Abnormal production of white blood cells is
    a. hemolytic
    b. leukemia
    c. thalassemia
    d. hemophilia
    e. none of the above

29. Blood poisoning is
    a. septicemia
    b. malaria
    c. thalassemia
    d. anemia
    e. none of the above

30. The Epstein-Barr virus causes
    a. septicemia
    b. malaria
    c. infectious mononucleosis
    d. sickle cell anemia
    e. none of the above

CHAPTER 14   THE CARDIOVASCULAR SYSTEM

CHAPTER OBJECTIVES

After studying this chapter, you should be able to:

1. Describe how the heart is positioned in the thoracic cavity.
2. List and describe the layers of the heart wall.
3. Name the chambers of the heart and their valves.
4. Name the major vessels that enter and exit the heart.
5. Describe blood flow through the heart.
6. Explain how the conduction system of the heart controls proper blood flow.
7. Describe the stages of a cardiac cycle.
8. Compare the anatomy of a vein, artery and capillary.
9. Name the major blood circulatory routes.

ACTIVITIES

A. COMPLETION

Fill in the blank spaces with the correct term.

1. The cardiovascular system consists of the _____ and the
   _____ _____.

2. _____ assist in the chemical reaction within cells.

3. Oxygen and nutrients from digested food help make the chemical energy _____.

4. Most of the heart is on the _____ side of the body's midline.

5. The membrane surrounding the heart is the _____ _____.

6. The outer layer of the membrane is the _____ _____, and the inferior
   inner layer is the _____ _____.

7. The outer layer of the heart is the _____.

8. The middle layer of the heart is the _____.

9. The inner layer of the heart is the _____.

10. The upper chambers of the heart are called the _____.

11. The lower chambers of the heart are called the _____.

12. The heart is separated into left and right sides by a _____.

13. The three veins supplying blood to the right atrium are the _____ and
    _____ venae cavae and the _____ _____.

14. In the lungs, blood gives up _____ _____ and receives _____.

15. The heart muscle is supplied with blood by the _____.

16. The descending aorta becomes the _____ aorta.

17. Of the four heart chambers, the _____ _____ has the thickest walls.

18. There are _____ valves in the heart and these are the _____, _____, _____ _____ and the _____ _____.

19. All of the valves have three cusps except the _____, which has _____ cusps.

20. The superior vena cava drains the _____ portion of the body, and the inferior vena cava the _____ portion.

21. Deoxygenated blood is _____ _____, whereas oxygenated blood is _____ _____.

22. The conduction system of the heart is actually a(n) _____ system.

23. The sinoatrial node (SA) is known as the _____.

24. The atrioventricular bundle is also known as the _____ of _____.

25. The actual contractions of the ventricles are stimulated by _____ _____.

26. Regulation of the beats of the heart reside in the _____ _____ system.

27. Contraction of the heart is the _____, and the relaxation phase is the _____.

28. Blood supply to the heart is via the _____ _____ route.

29. The one temporary circulatory route is _____ _____.

30. The three layers of blood vessels are the _____, _____ and the _____.

31. _____ are small arteries.

32. _____ are small veins.

33. _____ are vessels consisting of a single cell layer.

34. The first branch of the aortic arch is the _____ artery.

35. The _____ arteries supply the head, neck and brain.

B. MATCHING

Match the term on the right with the definition on the left.

Arteries

36. _____ divides into vertebral, axillary and brachial arteries

37. _____ 10 pairs

38. _____ supply the lungs

39. _____ phrenic

40. _____ left gastric, splenic, common hepatic

41. _____ right and left renal

42. _____ muscles of the abdomen

43. _____ femoral, popliteal, tibial, dorsal pedis

a. celiac trunk

b. kidneys

c. diaphragm

d. bronchial

e. internal iliac

f. intercostal

g. left subclavian

h. lumbar

Veins

44. _____ drains the forearm

45. _____ connects to the axillary

46. _____ where blood is drawn

47. _____ drains the thorax

48. _____ drains the calf and foot

49. _____ merge with the femoral

50. _____ drains the pelvis

51. _____ drains the liver

52. _____ drains the digestive tract

a. peroneal

b. azygos

c. hepatic

d. radius and ulna

e. external and internal iliac

f. cephalic

g. median cubital

h. saphenous

i. hepatic portal

General

53. _____ chest pain

54. _____ coronary thrombosis

55. _____ does not pump enough blood

56. _____ heart disease present at birth

a. heart failure

b. congenital

c. angina pectoris

d. blood clot

C. KEY TERMS

Use the text to look up the following terms. Write the definition or explanation.

57. Anastomosis: _____

_____

58. Anterior interventricular sulcus: _____

_____

59. Arch of the aorta: _____

_____

60. Atherosclerosis: _____

_____

61. Auricle: _____

_____

62. Cephalic vein: _____

_____

63. Chordae tendinae: _____

_____

64. Conduction myofibers: _____

_____

65. Coronary sulcus: _____

_____

66. Diastole: _____

_____

67. Hepatic portal circulation: _____

_____

68. Interventricular septum: _____

_____

69. Lumen: _____

_____

70. Musculi pectinati: _____

_____

71. Pacemaker: _____

_____

72. Papillary muscles: _____

_____

73. Pericardial fluid: _____

_____

74. Pulmonary circulation: _____

_____

75. Pulmonary semilunar valve: _____

_____

76. Right and left bundle branches: _____

_____

77. Serous pericardium: _____

_____

78. Systemic circulation: _____

_____

79. Systole: _____

_____

80. Trabeculae corneae: _____

_____

81. Vascular: _____

_____

D. LABELING EXERCISE

82. Label the chambers, vessels, valves and septum of the heart as indicated in Figure 14-1.

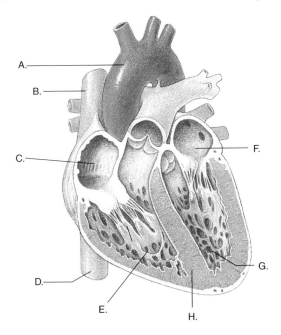

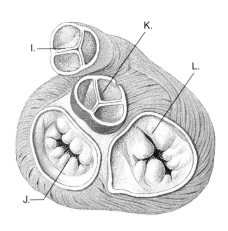

a. _____

b. _____

c. _____

d. _____

e. _____

f. _____

g. _____

h. _____

i. _____

j. _____

k. _____

l. _____

83. Label the arteries as indicated in Figure 14-2.

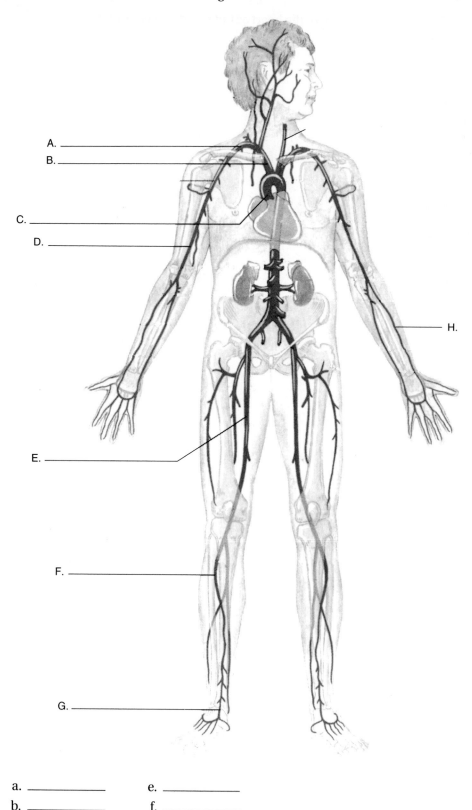

A. _____

B. _____

C. _____

D. _____

E. _____

F. _____

G. _____

H. _____

a. _____   e. _____

b. _____   f. _____

c. _____   g. _____

d. _____   h. _____

84. Label the veins indicated in Figure 14-3.

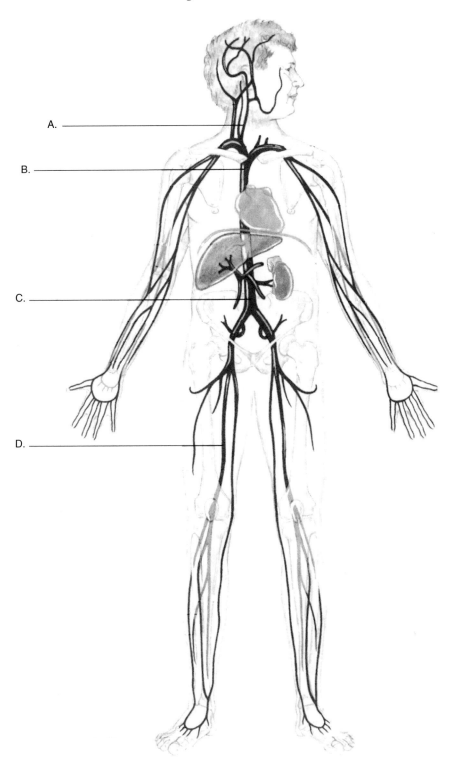

A. _____

B. _____

C. _____

D. _____

a. _____
b. _____
c. _____
d. _____

E. COLORING EXERCISE

85. Using Figure 14-4, color the veins blue and the arteries red.

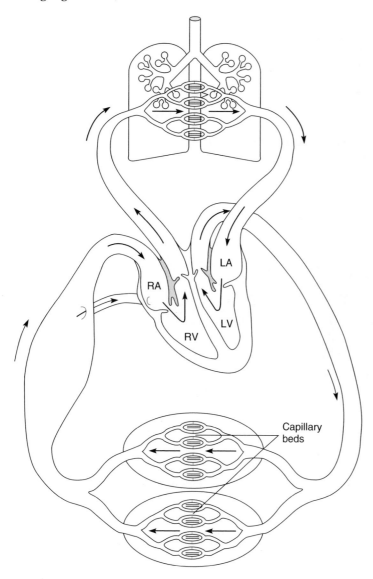

F. CRITICAL THINKING

Answer the following questions in complete sentences.

86. Given a blood pressure reading of 130/86, which is the systole and which is the diastole?

87. If a person has angina pectoris and is probably having an MI, explain what may be happening to the heart.

88. Why is the saphenous vein used for heart bypass surgery?

89. How does the cardiovascular system integrate with the skin to control body temperature?

90. Why do our muscles tire during exercise?

91. How does the lymphatic system work with the cardiovascular system to protect the body?

92. Why does the blood not flow backward in our veins?

93. What does adrenalin do to our cardiovascular system?

94. How does the conduction system control proper blood flow?

95. Why does cardiac output of a 70-year-old person often decrease by 75%?

96. Why is walking one of the best exercises to maintain good heart performance?

97. Distinguish among a cardiovascular technologist, an electrocardiographic technician and a cardiac sonographer.

G. CROSSWORD PUZZLE

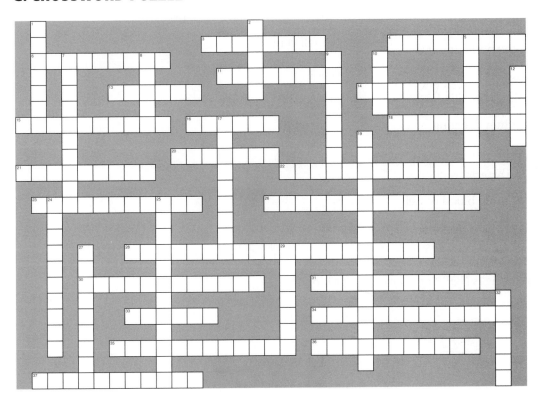

Complete the crossword puzzle using the following clues.

ACROSS

3. Another name for the mitral valve

4. SA node

6. 3-cusp valve regulating blood flow

11. Abnormal narrowing of the heart valve

13. Upper heart chamber

14. Relaxation phase of a heartbeat

DOWN

1. Contraction phase of a heartbeat

2. Hollow core of a blood vessel

5. Small artery

7. Cardiac muscle layer

8. Largest artery

9. Hormone promoting female vascular health

ACROSS

15. Three veins that send blood to the right atrium

16. Carries oxygenated blood from the heart

18. Lower heart chamber

20. External appendage of the atrium

21. Smallest blood vessel

22. Supplies blood to the lungs

23. Thigh vein draining into the inferior vena cava

26. Subclavian artery

28. Heart attack

30. Inflammation of the pericardium

31. High blood pressure

33. Organ supplied by the renal arteries

34. Helps maintain kidney function

35. Hole in the interatrial septum

36. Middle layer of the arterial wall

37. Junction of two or more blood vessels

DOWN

10. Returns deoxygenated blood to the heart

12. Help protect CV organs

17. Valve between the right atrium and right ventricle

19. Arterial disease caused by plaque buildup

24. Outermost layer of heart

25. Inflammation of the inner heart layer

27. Longest vein

29. Area of damaged cardiac tissue

32. Small vein

CHAPTER QUIZ

1. Which of the following is NOT transported by the blood?
   a. oxygen
   b. urine
   c. hormones
   d. waste
   e. nutrients

2. The normal heartbeat is about how many times per minute?
   a. 60
   b. 100
   c. 90
   d. 72
   e. none of the above

3. The heart is composed primarily of
   a. fat
   b. blood
   c. lymph
   d. muscle
   e. cartilage

4. The serous pericardium is known as what layer of the pericardial sac?
   a. fibrous
   b. intima
   c. parietal
   d. visceral
   e. precordial

5. The epicardium can also be referred to as the
   a. parietal pericardium
   b. pericardial cavity
   c. visceral peritoneum
   d. parietal peritoneum
   e. serous peritoneum

6. The endocardium is made up of which type of tissue?
   a. epithelial
   b. connective
   c. muscle
   d. osseus
   e. none of the above

7. The atrial appendage similar to a dog's ear is the
   a. auricle
   b. trabeculae
   c. septum
   d. bicuspid
   e. tricuspid

8. The right atrium receives blood from all parts of the body except the
   a. brain
   b. hands
   c. kidneys
   d. liver
   e. lungs

9. The superior vena cava is also known as the
   a. small vena cava
   b. pulmonary vein
   c. posterior vena cava
   d. anterior vena cava
   e. coronary sinus

10. The smallest of the four heart chambers is the
    a. right atrium
    b. left atrium
    c. right ventricle
    d. left ventricle
    e. coronary sinus

11. The only heart valve with two cusps is the
    a. tricuspid
    b. mitral
    c. pulmonary
    d. aortic
    e. semilunar

12. Blood receives oxygen in the
    a. liver
    b. kidneys
    c. lungs
    d. heart
    e. pancreas

13. Blood deposits which of the following in the lungs?
    a. oxygen
    b. urine
    c. hormones
    d. carbon dioxide
    e. renin

14. Blood from the lungs returns to the heart through how many veins?
    a. 2
    b. 4
    c. 6
    d. 8
    e. 3

15. Blood from the lungs returns to which of the following?
    a. right ventricle
    b. left ventricle
    c. right atrium
    d. left atrium
    e. superior vena cava

16. Increase or decrease in heart rate is controlled by which part of the nervous system?
    a. central
    b. autonomic
    c. peripheral
    d. forebrain
    e. temporal

17. Contraction of the ventricles is stimulated by the
    a. SA node
    b. AV node
    c. bundle branches
    d. Bundle of His
    e. Purkinje's fibers

18. A cardiac cycle consists of contractions of
    a. both atria
    b. an atrium and a ventricle
    c. two ventricles
    d. two atria then two ventricles
    e. all four chambers at once

19. A complete cycle of blood flow is called
    a. pulmonary circulation
    b. coronary circulation
    c. hepatic portal circulation
    d. cerebral circulation
    e. systemic circulation

20. Two major properties of arteries are
    a. irritability/contractility
    b. thickness/irritability
    c. hollowness/thinness
    d. elasticity/contractility
    e. anastomosis/fragility

21. Which vessels have walls one cell thick?
    a. venules
    b. arteries
    c. capillaries
    d. arterioles
    e. veins

22. Veins have something that arteries do not. Which of the following is it?
    a. irritability
    b. valves
    c. junctions
    d. smooth muscle
    e. contractility

23. When the aorta arches and begins descending down along the spine, then goes through the diaphragm, it is known as the
    a. abdominal aorta
    b. thoracic aorta
    c. subclavian artery
    d. esophageal artery
    e. brachiocephalic artery

24. The left common carotid artery branches from the
    a. right common carotid artery
    b. aortic arch
    c. left subclavian artery
    d. thoracic artery
    e. axillary artery

25. The final branches of the abdominal aorta are the
    a. popliteal arteries
    b. femoral arteries
    c. common iliac arteries
    d. tibial arteries
    e. inferior mesenteric arteries

26. Veins that drain the arm include all of the following EXCEPT the
    a. brachial
    b. cephalic
    c. vertebral
    d. basilic
    e. median cubital

27. All of the following veins drain into the superior vena cava EXCEPT the
    a. internal jugular
    b. azygos
    c. internal iliac
    d. vertebral
    e. subclavian

28. Which of the following does not drain into the inferior vena cava?
    a. azygos
    b. hepatic portal
    c. saphenous
    d. gonadal
    e. popliteal

29. Which of the following is NOT an inflammatory condition?
    a. endocarditis
    b. atherosclerosis
    c. pericarditis
    d. gastritis
    e. myocarditis

30. Two common congenital heart defects are
    a. thrombosis/angina
    b. hypertension/septal defect
    c. stenotic heart valves/hypertension
    d. angina/stenotic heart valves
    e. septal defect/stenotic heart valves

CHAPTER 15   THE LYMPHATIC SYSTEM

CHAPTER OBJECTIVES

After studying this chapter, you should be able to:

1. Name the functions of the lymphatic system.
2. Explain what lymph is and how it forms.
3. Describe lymph flow through the body.
4. Name the principal lymphatic trunks.
5. Describe the functions of the tonsils and spleen.
6. Explain the unique role the thymus gland plays as part of the lymphatic system.
7. Describe the different types of immunity.
8. Explain the difference between blood and the lymphatic capillaries.
9. Explain the difference between active and passive immunity.
10. Define an *antigen* and an *antibody*.

ACTIVITIES

A. COMPLETION

Fill in the blank spaces with the correct term.

1. The four organs of the lymph system are the _____, _____, _____ and the _____ _____.

2. Interstitial fluid is _____ forced from capillaries.

3. Edema is another name for _____.

4. _____ is interstitial fluid that has entered a lymphatic capillary.

5. Chyle looks milky because of its _____ content.

6. The larger lymph vessels are the _____.

7. The larger lymph vessels of the viscera generally follow the routes of _____.

8. Efferent lymphatic vessels leave the lymph nodes at the _____.

9. Trabeculae are _____ _____.

10. Those vessels entering a lymph node are the _____ lymphatic vessels.

11. The lymph nodule surrounds a _____ _____, which produces lymphocytes.

12. The stroma of a lymph node is made up of the _____, the _____ and the _____.

13. In the lymph node, any microorganisms or foreign substances stimulate _____ to divide, thereby activating the _____ _____.

14. Lymph trunks are formed by uniting _____ vessels.

15. The principal trunks pass their lymph into the _____ _____ and the _____ _____ _____.

16. The lymph flow cycle is completed when the lymph is drained back into the _____.

17. The _____ tonsils are the ones removed in a tonsillectomy.

18. The adenoids are the _____ tonsils.

19. The bilobed mass of tissue located in the mediastinum is the _____ _____.

20. In the spleen, _____ of worn-out red blood cells releases hemoglobin.

21. Peyer's patches are found in the wall of the _____ _____.

22. The _____ of the Peyer's patches destroy bacteria.

23. Disease-causing microorganisms are called _____.

24. Plasma cells come from _____ _____.

25. High molecular weight proteins are the _____.

26. The body's production of antibodies against an antigen is _____ immunity.

27. The type of immunity received by the fetus from the mother is _____.

28. _____ _____ _____ destroy virus-invaded body cells.

29. _____ _____ is the disease of the lymphatic system with historical implications.

30. _____ is a tumor of the lymphatic system.

B. MATCHING

Match the term on the right with the definition on the left.

31. _____ lymph organs   a. lymphocytes

32. _____ interstitial fluid originally   b. tonsillectomy

33. _____ lymph vessels in villi   c. B lymphocytes

34. _____ chyle   d. bubonic plague

35. _____ aggregation of nodes   e. lymph trunk

36. _____ capsular extension   f. Peyer's patches

37. _____ lymph sinuses   g. milky lymph

38. _____ germinal centers   h. plasma

39. _____ efferent vessel union   i. tonsils

40. _____ pharyngeal tonsils   j. trabeculae

41. _____ palatine tonsils removed   k. lymphoma

42. _____ aggregate lymph follicles   l. groin

43. _____ provide humoral immunity   m. spaces

44. _____ lymph tissue tumor   n. lacteals

45. _____ *Klebsiella pestis*   o. adenoids

C. KEY TERMS

Use the text to look up the following terms. Write the definition or explanation.

46. Active immunity: _____

_____

47. Antibodies/immunoglobulins: _____

_____

48. Antigen: _____

_____

49. Cellular immunity: _____

_____

50. Complement: _____

_____

51. Germinal center: _____

_____

52. Helper T cells: _____

_____

53. Humoral immunity: _____

_____

54. Killer T cells: _____

_____

55. Lymph nodes/glands: _____

_____

56. Lymph sinus: _____

_____

57. Lymphokines: _____

_____

58. Memory cells: _____

_____

59. Passive immunity: _____

_____

60. Pathogens: _____

_____

61. Peyer's patches: _____

_____

62. Plasma cells: _____

_____

63. Suppressor T cells: _____

_____

64. T lymphocytes/T cells:_____

_____

65. Trabeculae: _____

_____

D. LABELING EXERCISE

66. Label the correct organs as indicated in Figure 15-1.

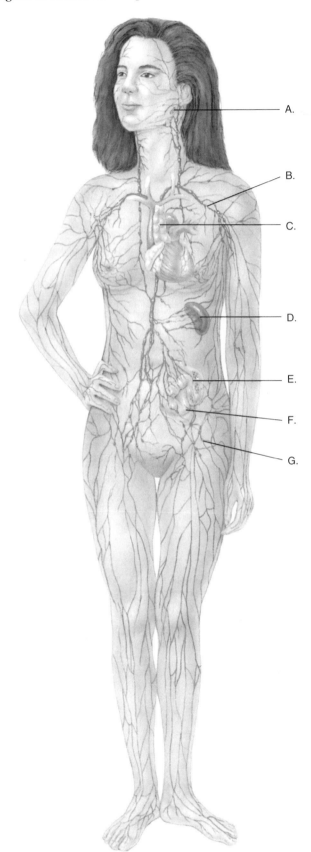

A.

B.

C.

D.

E.

F.

G.

a. _____

b. _____

c. _____

d. _____

e. _____

f. _____

g. _____

67. Label the correct lymph nodes as indicated in Figure 15-2.

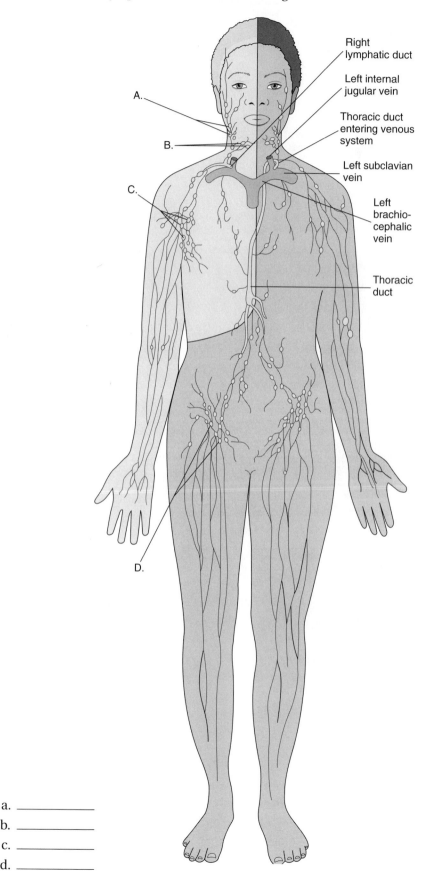

Right
lymphatic duct

Left internal
jugular vein

Thoracic duct
entering venous
system

Left subclavian
vein

Left
brachio-
cephalic
vein

Thoracic
duct

A.

B.

C.

D.

a. _____

b. _____

c. _____

d. _____

E. COLORING EXERCISE

68. Use Figure 15-3 to color the venule blue, the arteriole red, the blood capillary red, the lymphatic capillary green and the interstitial fluid yellow.

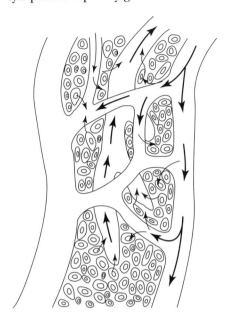

F. CRITICAL THINKING

Answer the following questions in complete sentences.

69. Why can lymph vessels transport larger molecules than blood vessels?

70. Describe the framework of the lymph node.

71. Explain the immune response in a lymph node.

72. Differentiate elephantiasis in Africa and in Malaysia.

73. How does removal of the spleen affect immunity?

74. What are antibodies and how do they work?

75. Why does acquired immunodeficiency syndrome (AIDS) cause death by opportunistic diseases?

76. Explain the effect of age-related changes in the lymphatic system.

77. Differentiate between an immunologist and an oncologist.

G. CROSSWORD PUZZLE

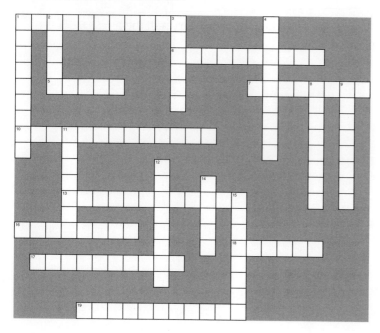

Complete the crossword puzzle using the following clues.

ACROSS

1. Engulf and digest antigens
5. Swelling
6. Large lymph vessels
7. Nodule of dense tissue in lymph node
10. Disease from blocked lymph system
13. Fluid found between tissue cells
16. Vessels entering lymph nodes
17. Enzymes that attack antigens
18. Formed by uniting efferent vessels
19. Chemical from T lymphocyte

DOWN

1. Chemicals released by macrophages
2. Lymph in lacteals
3. Single largest lymphatic tissue mass
4. Disease-causing microorganisms
8. Ability to resist infection
9. Pharyngeal tonsils
11. Immunity that is naturally conferred
12. Foreign proteins
14. Lymph node depression
15. Lymph vessels in intestinal villi

CHAPTER QUIZ

1. Which cells are formed by replicating B cells?

   a. helper T cells
   b. plasma cells
   c. memory cells
   d. suppressor T cells
   e. none of the above

2. Which cells exist in the body for years?
   a. helper T cells
   b. plasma cells
   c. memory cells
   d. suppressor T cells
   e. none of the above

3. Which cells engulf and digest antigens?
   a. helper T cells
   b. plasma cells
   c. memory cells
   d. suppressor T cells
   e. none of the above

4. Which cells bind with specific antigens presented by macrophages?
   a. helper T cells
   b. plasma cells
   c. memory cells
   d. suppressor T cells
   e. none of the above

5. Inflammation of the lymphatic vessels is called
   a. lymphoma
   b. lymphadenitis
   c. lymphangitis
   d. bubonic plague
   e. none of the above

6. The fluid that moves out of the blood capillaries is called
   a. lymph
   b. interstitial fluid
   c. plasma
   d. chyle
   e. none of the above

7. When that fluid is in the lacteals, it is called
   a. lymph
   b. interstitial fluid
   c. plasma
   d. chyle
   e. none of the above

8. Before the fluid leaves the blood capillaries, it is called
   a. lymph
   b. interstitial fluid
   c. plasma
   d. chyle
   e. none of the above

9. The oval to bean-shaped structures of the lymphatic system are the
   a. lacteals
   b. vessels
   c. glands
   d. trabeculae
   e. none of the above

10. The vessels entering a lymph node are the
    a. efferent
    b. trabeculae
    c. germinal
    d. afferent
    e. none of the above

11. The structure producing lymphocytes and surrounded by the lymph nodule is the
    a. efferent
    b. trabeculae
    c. germinal
    d. afferent
    e. none of the above

12. Which of the following helps make up the framework of the lymph node?
    a. efferent
    b. trabeculae
    c. germinal
    d. afferent
    e. none of the above

13. The hilum is which of the following?
    a. efferent
    b. trabeculae
    c. germinal
    d. afferent
    e. none of the above

14. The vessels which unite to form lymph trunks are the
    a. efferent
    b. trabeculae
    c. germinal
    d. afferent
    e. none of the above

15. Which of the following is NOT one of the body's lymphatic trunks?

    a. lumbar

    b. thoracic

    c. bronchomediastinal

    d. subclavian

    e. none of the above

16. Which of the following drains lymph from the lower extremities?

    a. lumbar

    b. thoracic

    c. bronchomediastinal

    d. subclavian

    e. none of the above

17. Which of the following is NOT a lymphatic trunk?

    a. thoracic

    b. jugular

    c. subclavian

    d. lumbar

    e. none of the above

18. When the lymph cycle is complete, the fluid goes back to the

    a. nodes

    b. ducts

    c. lungs

    d. blood

    e. none of the above

19. Which of the following are NOT tonsils?

    a. palatine

    b. adenoids

    c. lingual

    d. pharyngeal

    e. none of the above

20. Which of the following is NOT a lymph organ?

    a. tonsils

    b. spleen

    c. thymus

    d. Peyer's patches

    e. none of the above

21. The aggregated lymphatic follicles are the

    a. tonsils

    b. spleen

    c. thymus

    d. Peyer's patches

    e. none of the above

22. Immunity produced by the body's lymphoid tissue is
    a. passive
    b. inherited
    c. cellular
    d. injected
    e. none of the above

23. Which of the following gamma globulins activates complement?
    a. G
    b. A
    c. M
    d. D
    e. none of the above

24. Which of the following gamma globulins is important in B-cell activation?
    a. G
    b. A
    c. M
    d. D
    e. none of the above

25. Which of the following gamma globulins develops in blood plasma?
    a. G
    b. A
    c. M
    d. D
    e. none of the above

CHAPTER 16   NUTRITION AND THE DIGESTIVE SYSTEM

CHAPTER OBJECTIVES

After studying this chapter, you should be able to:

1. List and describe the five basic activities of the digestive process.
2. List the four layers or tunics of the walls of the digestive tract.
3. Name the major and accessory organs of the digestive tract and their component anatomic parts.
4. Explain the major digestive enzymes and how they function.
5. Explain the functions of the liver.
6. Explain how absorption of nutrients occurs in the small intestine and how the feces form in the large intestine.
7. Name and describe the functions of the organs of the digestive tract.

ACTIVITIES

A. COMPLETION

Fill in the blank spaces with the correct term.

1. Breaking down food into simpler substances that the cells can use is the process of _____.

2. Mastication is the process of _____.

3. _____ plus lipase plus water produces glycerol.

4. The digestion of food begins in the mouth through the action of the enzyme _____.

5. The lining of the entire alimentary canal has _____ layers or _____.

6. The tunica muscularis is responsible for propelling food along by _____.

7. The mesentery is an extension of the _____ _____.

8. The anterior part of the roof of the mouth is the _____ _____.

9. The lingual frenulum is a _____ dividing the tongue.

10. The tongue is supported by the _____ bone.

11. Saliva is mostly water, but an important chemical activator in it is _____.

12. If the mumps virus infects the pancreas, it can cause _____.

13. The _____ extend slightly into each tooth socket.

14. Infants' teeth are called _____ teeth.

15. Teeth can have as many as _____ root projections.

16. Tooth decay is also called _____ _____.

17. There are three parts to the pharynx; they are the _____, _____ and the _____.

18. The tube connecting the laryngopharynx and the stomach is the _____, which passes through the _____ and _____.

19. The stomach begins with the _____ and ends at the _____.

20. The small intestine begins with the _____ and ends with the _____.

21. An ulcer can be caused by either excess _____ or _____.

22. Alpha and beta cells of the pancreas secrete _____ and _____.

23. Another cell of the pancreas secretes enzymes; this is the _____.

24. There are _____ major functions of the liver.

25. The functions of the gallbladder are _____ and _____.

26. The walls of the small intestine are protected from digestion by _____.

27. The folds of the small intestine are called _____, and the projections are called _____.

28. The bowel begins with the _____ and ends at the _____ _____.

29. The end of the alimentary canal is the _____.

30. The final act of the digestive system is _____.

31. Hepatitis can be caused by virus _____ or virus _____.

32. Gallstones are caused by _____.

33. A chronic, inflammatory bowel disease with unknown origin is _____ _____.

34. Diverticulosis is a disorder characterized by _____ in the muscular layer of the colon.

35. Inflammation and enlargement of rectal veins is _____.

B. MATCHING

Match the term on the right with the definition on the left.

36. _____ degenerative liver disease

37. _____ inflammatory bowel disease

38. _____ rectal vein enlargement

39. _____ digested food to the cardiovascular system

40. _____ gastrointestinal tract

41. _____ visceral peritoneum

42. _____ posterior roof of the mouth

43. _____ septum divides the tongue

44. _____ important in licking

45. _____ salivary enzyme

46. _____ premolar

47. _____ three cusps

a. lingual frenulum

b. sigmoid colon

c. bicuspids

d. amylase

e. filiform papillae

f. cecum

g. pepsinogen

h. fundus

i. jejunum

j. pancreatic duct

k. soft palate

l. Crohn's disease

48. _____ enamel covered

49. _____ tube behind the trachea

50. _____ rounded portion above the cardia

51. _____ principal gastric enzyme

52. _____ duct of Wirsung

53. _____ second portion of the large intestine

54. _____ first part of the large intestine

55. _____ colon joins the rectum

m. absorption

n. esophagus

o. hemorrhoids

p. cirrhosis

q. tricuspid

r. tunica serosa

s. crown

t. alimentary canal

C. KEY TERMS

Use the text to look up the following terms. Write the definition or explanation.

56. Absorption: _____

_____

57. Amylase: _____

_____

58. Apical foramen: _____

_____

59. Brunner's glands/duodenal glands: _____

_____

60. Cardia: _____

_____

61. Cementum: _____

_____

62. Chyme: _____

_____

63. Circumvallate papillae: _____

_____

64. Crypt of Lieberkuhn: _____

_____

65. Diarrhea: _____

_____

66. Digestion: _____

_____

67. Esophageal hiatus: _____

_____

68. Falciform ligament: _____

_____

69. Fungiform papillae: _____

_____

70. Hard palate: _____

_____

71. Haustrae: _____

_____

72. Ileocecal valve: _____

_____

73. Kupffer's cells: _____

_____

74. Mediastinum: _____

_____

75. Microvilli/brushborder: _____

_____

76. Muscularis mucosa: _____

_____

77. Parietal cells: _____

_____

78. Pepsin: _____

_____

79. Pepsinogen: _____

_____

80. Peristalsis: _____

_____

81. Plicae: _____

_____

82. Right colic (hepatic) flexure: _____

_____

83. Rugae: _____

_____

84. Uvula: _____

_____

85. Zymogenic/chief cells: _____

_____

D. LABELING EXERCISE

86. Label the parts of the digestive system as indicated in Figure 16-1.

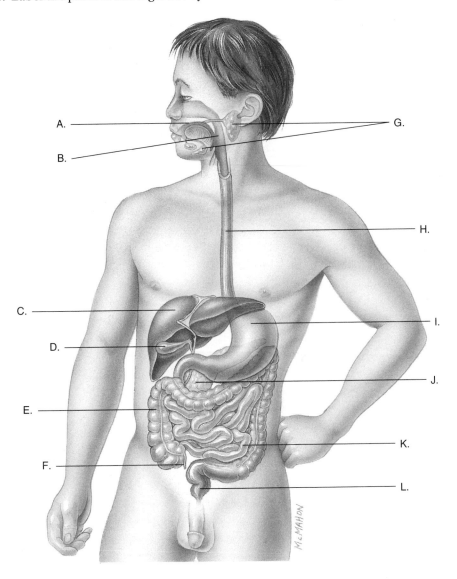

A. _____

B. _____

C. _____

D. _____

E. _____

F. _____

G. _____

H. _____

I. _____

J. _____

K. _____

L. _____

a. _____

b. _____

c. _____

d. _____

e. _____

f. _____

g. _____

h. _____

i. _____

j. _____

k. _____

l. _____

87. Label the parts of the stomach and the small intestine as indicated in Figure 16-2.

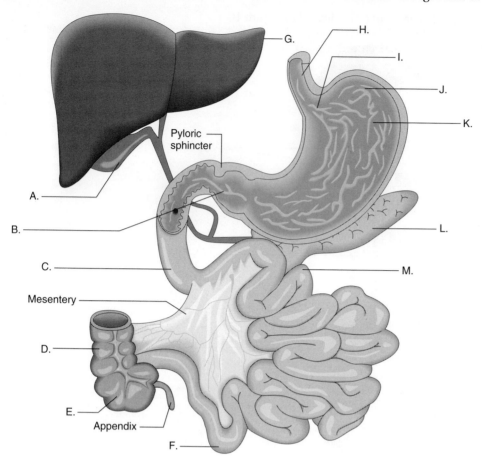

a. _____

b. _____

c. _____

d. _____

e. _____

f. _____

g. _____

h. _____

i. _____

j. _____

k. _____

l. _____

m. _____

E. COLORING EXERCISE

88. Using Figure 16-3, color the ascending colon red, the transverse colon green, the descending colon yellow, the sigmoid colon brown, the rectum orange and the cecum blue.

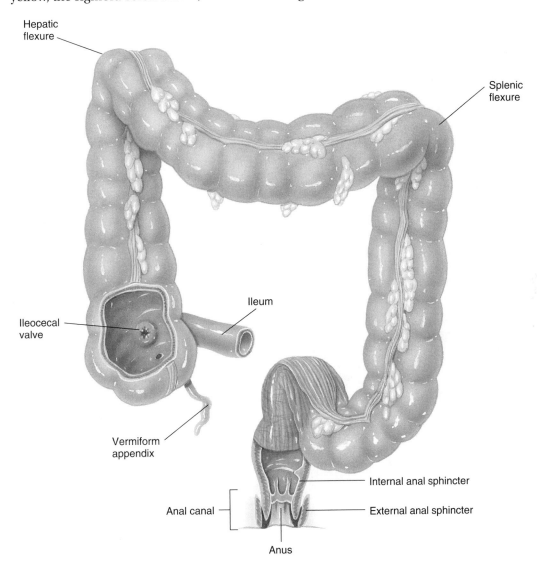

F. CRITICAL THINKING

Answer the following questions in complete sentences.

89. Why do cavities occur?

90. Explain the first stage of digestion.

91. Why does food stuck in the esophagus cause breathing difficulties?

92. Why does a hiatal hernia cause a burning sensation in the esophagus?

93. Explain the formation of an ulcer.

94. Incomplete development of the hard palate (cleft palate) causes nasality. Why?

95. How does the pancreas contribute to the digestive process?

96. Explain absorption in the small intestine.

97. As people age, why do they become more susceptible to digestive system disorders?

98. Of the career opportunities presented, choose one that is the most interesting to you. Explain why.

G. CROSSWORD PUZZLE

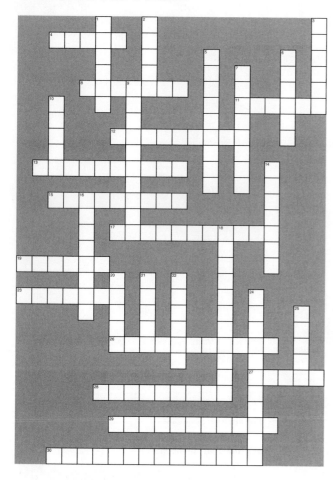

Complete the crossword puzzle using the following clues.

ACROSS

4. One of the largest organs of the system

8. Anticoagulant

11. Tooth that tears food

12. Inflammation of the liver

13. Waste elimination

15. Breakdown of food

17. Stores bile

19. Teeth are made of it

23. Breaks down starch in the mouth

DOWN

1. Teeth

2. Tooth that grinds food

3. Folds of the intestine

5. Extension of the visceral peritoneum

6. 99.5% H_2O

7. Teeth that cut food

9. Tunica serosa

10. Semifluid in the intestine

14. Connects with the duodenum

ACROSS

26. Chewing

27. Stomach folds

28. Taking in food

29. Pushing food along

30. Pouchlike herniation

DOWN

16. Gums

18. Swallowing

20. First part of large intestine

21. Disease of the salivary glands

22. Between the crown and root

24. Enlarged rectal veins

25. Hangs from the palate

CHAPTER QUIZ

1. An inflammation of the liver that can be caused by alcohol or a virus is called
   a. cirrhosis
   b. Crohn's disease
   c. hepatitis
   d. diverticulosis
   e. none of the above

2. When the liver becomes scarred and degenerates, it is called
   a. cirrhosis
   b. Crohn's disease
   c. hepatitis
   d. diverticulosis
   e. none of the above

3. A chronic, inflammatory bowel disease is called
   a. cirrhosis
   b. Crohn's disease
   c. hepatitis
   d. diverticulosis
   e. none of the above

4. When the bowel has pouchlike herniations, it is called
   a. cirrhosis
   b. Crohn's disease
   c. hepatitis
   d. diverticulosis
   e. none of the above

5. The movement of food through the alimentary canal by smooth muscles is called
   a. ingestion
   b. digestion
   c. mastication
   d. peristalsis
   e. none of the above

6. Taking food into the body is called
    a. ingestion
    b. digestion
    c. mastication
    d. peristalsis
    e. none of the above

7. The act of swallowing is called
    a. deglutition
    b. mastication
    c. ingestion
    d. peristalsis
    e. none of the above

8. Which of the following is NOT an accessory structure of the gastrointestinal tract?
    a. teeth
    b. tongue
    c. liver
    d. salivary glands
    e. none of the above

9. Which of the following is NOT one of the four tunics of the alimentary canal?
    a. tunica mucosa
    b. lamina propria
    c. muscularis
    d. serosa
    e. none of the above

10. Which of the papillae are important in licking?
    a. fungiform
    b. circumvallate
    c. filiform
    d. frenulum
    e. none of the above

11. The salivary glands that secrete the least amount of saliva are the
    a. parotids
    b. submandibular
    c. buccal
    d. sublingual
    e. none of the above

12. Which of the following substances is NOT found in saliva?
    a. amylase
    b. urea
    c. lipase
    d. phosphates
    e. none of the above

13. The number of permanent teeth is
    a. 20
    b. 13
    c. 24
    d. 32
    e. none of the above

14. Cavities are known as
    a. dentes
    b. gingivae
    c. pulp
    d. caries
    e. none of the above

15. Which of the following are NOT teeth?
    a. molar
    b. canine
    c. incisor
    d. cuspid
    e. none of the above

16. All of the following are parts of the pharynx EXCEPT
    a. tracheo
    b. naso
    c. oro
    c. laryngo
    e. none of the above

17. The major symptom of a hiatal hernia is
    a. tickling
    b. raspy
    c. burning
    d. pressure
    e. none of the above

18. All of the following are parts of the stomach EXCEPT
    a. cardia
    b. fundus
    c. pylorus
    d. antrum
    e. none of the above

19. All of the following are secretion cells of the stomach EXCEPT
    a. zymogenic
    b. alpha
    c. parietal
    d. mucous
    e. none of the above

20. The folds of the stomach are called
    a. pepsin
    b. HCl
    c. rugae
    d. pepsinogen
    e. none of the above

21. Approximately 80% of nutrient absorption takes place in the
    a. stomach
    b. small intestine
    c. large intestine
    d. liver
    e. none of the above

22. Digestion of protein begins in the
    a. stomach
    b. pancreas
    c. liver
    d. large intestine
    e. none of the above

23. Which of the following is NOT a function of the liver?
    a. produce heparin
    b. phagocytose blood cells
    c. detoxify
    d. produce bile salts
    e. none of the above

24. All of the following are sections of the small intestine EXCEPT
    a. duodenum
    b. cecum
    c. jejunum
    d. ileum
    e. none of the above

25. The absorption structures of the small intestine are
    a. villi
    b. plicae
    c. chyme
    d. rugae
    e. none of the above

26. The valves of the alimentary canal are of which type?
    a. flap
    b. cusp
    c. bicusp
    d. sphincter
    e. none of the above

27. All of the following are movements that occur in the large intestine EXCEPT
    a. haustral churning
    b. peristalsis
    c. mass peristalsis
    d. vibration
    e. none of the above

28. Which of the following is NOT a part of the colon?
    a. rectum
    b. ascending
    c. sigmoid
    d. transverse
    e. none of the above

29. Which of the following is NOT a function of the large intestine?
    a. water absorption
    b. feces formation
    c. vitamin production
    d. mucus production
    e. none of the above

30. Which of the following is the end of the alimentary canal?
    a. sigmoid
    b. rectum
    c. anus
    d. descending colon
    e. none of the above

CHAPTER 17   THE RESPIRATORY SYSTEM

CHAPTER OBJECTIVES

After studying this chapter, you should be able to:

1. Explain the function of the respiratory system.
2. Name the organs of the system.
3. Define the parts of the internal nose and their functions.
4. Name the three areas of the pharynx and explain their anatomy.
5. Name the cartilages and membranes of the larynx and how they function.
6. Explain how the anatomy of the trachea prevents collapse during breathing and allows for esophageal expansion during swallowing.
7. Explain what is meant by the term *bronchial tree*.
8. Describe the structure and function of the lungs and pleura.
9. Describe the overall process of gas exchange in the lungs and tissues.
10. Define *ventilation*, *external respiration* and *internal respiration*.

ACTIVITIES

A. COMPLETION

Fill in the blank spaces with the correct term.

1. There are two systems responsible for supplying oxygen and eliminating carbon dioxide; they are the _____ and the _____ systems.
2. The bridge of the nose is formed by the _____ bones.
3. The underside of the external nose has two openings called _____.
4. Posteriorly, the internal nose connects with the _____.
5. The nasal septum divides the left and right _____ _____.
6. The interior structures of the nose have _____ functions.
7. Olfactory receptors are located in the membrane of the _____ meatus.
8. The adenoid tonsils are located in the posterior wall of the _____ _____.
9. The opening of the oropharynx is called the _____.
10. The voice box is the _____.
11. The epiglottis forms a lid over the _____.
12. The paired rod-shaped cartilage structures of the larynx are the _____.
13. The false vocal cords are the _____ _____.
14. The goblet cells of the trachea produce _____.
15. There are 16 to 20 incomplete rings of _____ cartilage in the trachea.
16. The lobar bronchi are the _____ bronchi, and the segmental bronchi are the _____ bronchi.

17. The pleural membrane covering the wall of the cavity is the _____ , and the membrane covering the lungs is the _____ .

18. The air sacs where gas exchange takes place are the _____ .

19. Movement of air between the atmosphere and the lungs is called _____ .

20. Internal respiration is the exchange of gases between the blood and _____ .

21. _____ _____ affects the secretory cells of the lungs.

22. Any infection in the lungs is known as _____ .

23. Whooping cough is also known as _____ .

24. The disease caused by excessive exposure to asbestos, silica or coal dust is _____ _____ .

25. Bronchitis causes a swelling of the _____ _____ .

B. MATCHING

Match the term on the right with the definition on the left.

26. _____ food convert to ATP

27. _____ internal nose to pharynx

28. _____ separates nasal cavities

29. _____ sense of smell

30. _____ another name for auditory tubes

31. _____ passage for food and air

32. _____ single piece in the larynx

33. _____ Adam's apple

34. _____ leaf-shaped cartilage

35. _____ paired, cone-shaped

36. _____ false vocal cords

37. _____ true vocal cords

38. _____ primary bronchi divide into

39. _____ segmented bronchi

40. _____ enclose and protect the lungs

41. _____ space between the membranes

42. _____ gases diffuse through it

43. _____ exchange gas between blood cells

44. _____ cavities inside the nostrils

45. _____ affects the secretion cells of the lungs

a. epiglottis

b. oropharynx

c. cystic fibrosis

d. thyroid cartilage

e. vocal folds

f. pleural membrane

g. tertiary bronchi

h. corniculate cartilage

i. internal respiration

j. cricoid cartilage

k. nasal septum

l. lobar bronchi

m. olfactory stimuli

n. respiratory membrane

o. eustachian tubes

p. cellular respiration

q. internal nares

r. pleural cavity

s. vestibules

t. vestibular folds

C. KEY TERMS

Use the text to look up the following terms. Write the definition or explanation.

46. Alveolar-capillary membrane/respiratory membrane: _____

_____

47. Alveolar ducts/atria: _____

_____

48. Alveolar sacs: _____

_____

49. Arytenoid cartilages: _____

_____

50. Bronchopulmonary segment: _____

_____

51. Epiglottis: _____

_____

52. External respiration: _____

_____

53. Fauces: _____

_____

54. Glottis: _____

_____

55. Inferior meatus: _____

_____

56. Internal nares: _____

_____

57. Internal respiration: _____

_____

58. Larynx: _____

_____

59. Lobules: _____

_____

60. Middle meatus: _____

_____

61. Nasopharynx: _____

_____

62. Olfactory stimuli: _____

_____

63. Parietal pleura: _____

_____

64. Partial pressure: _____

_____

65. Superior meatus: _____

_____

66. Surfactant: _____

_____

67. Trachea: _____

_____

68. Ventilation/breathing: _____

_____

69. Visceral pleura: _____

_____

D. LABELING EXERCISE

70. Label the parts of the respiratory system as indicated in Figure 17-1.

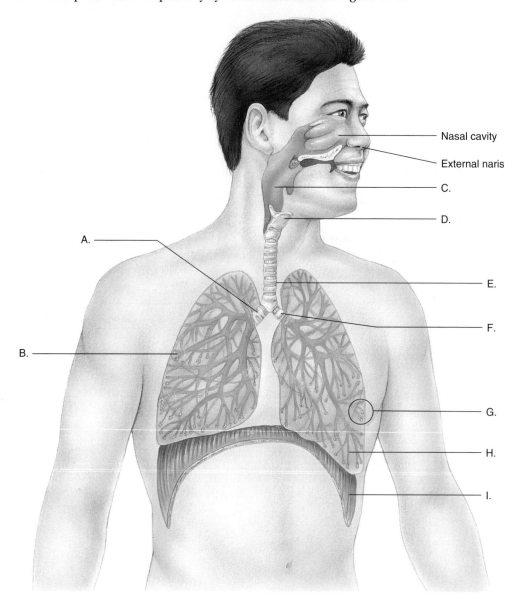

Nasal cavity

External naris

C.

D.

A.

E.

B.

F.

G.

H.

I.

a. _____
b. _____
c. _____
d. _____
e. _____
f. _____
g. _____
h. _____
i. _____

71. Label the parts of the nasal cavity and pharynx as indicated in Figure 17-2.

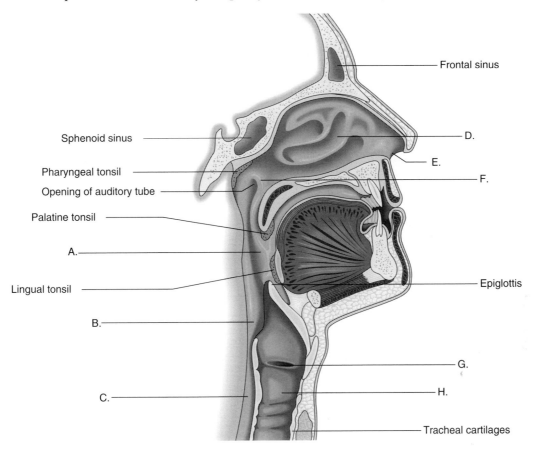

Frontal sinus

Sphenoid sinus

D.

E.

Pharyngeal tonsil

F.

Opening of auditory tube

Palatine tonsil

A.

Lingual tonsil

Epiglottis

B.

G.

H.

C.

Tracheal cartilages

a. _____

b. _____

c. _____

d. _____

e. _____

f. _____

g. _____

h. _____

E. COLORING EXERCISE

72. Using Figure 17-3, color the hyoid bone green, the larynx red, the lungs blue and the primary bronchi orange.

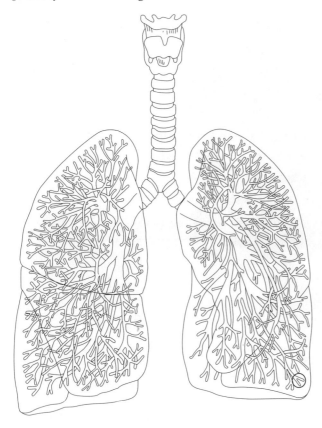

F. CRITICAL THINKING

Answer the following questions in complete sentences.

73. How is the nose the first line of defense against foreign material?

74. How does material inadvertently enter the trachea?

75. What are the functions of the C rings of cartilage in the trachea?

76. Why is it called the "bronchial tree"?

77. Explain emphysema.

78. How do the nervous system and the respiratory system assist each other?

79. Explain fetal respiration.

80. What effect will age-related changes have on the respiratory system?

81. Using an online reference, identify the types of activities performed by a respiratory therapist.

G. CROSSWORD PUZZLE

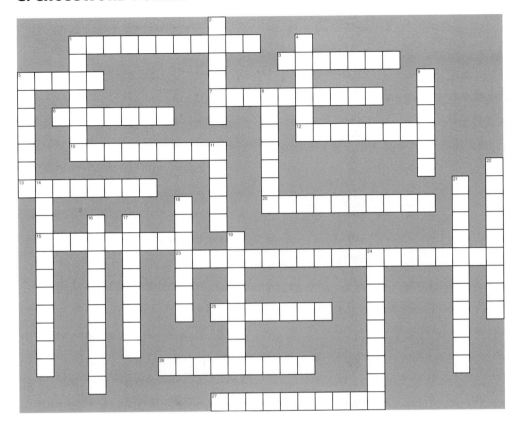

Complete the crossword puzzle using the following clues.

ACROSS

1. Cone-shaped cartilage
3. Adam's apple cartilage
5. Alveolar ducts
6. Many small compartments
7. Covers glottis
10. Breathing muscle
12. Segmented bronchi
13. Carries oxygen
15. Lung infection
20. Prevents collapse of alveoli
23. Converts food to ATP
25. Tubes from the trachea to the lungs
26. Destruction of alveoli walls
27. Anterior nasal cavities

DOWN

1. Cartilage of larynx
2. Opening of oropharynx
4. Pharynx
5. Air sacs
8. Space between vocal cords
9. Voice box
11. Shelf passageways
14. Exchange of gases
16. Nasal cavity bones
17. External nares
18. Windpipe
19. Pleuritis
21. Breathing
22. Ladle-shaped cartilage
24. Whooping cough

CHAPTER QUIZ

1. Along with the respiratory system, which system has the responsibility of supplying oxygen and eliminating carbon dioxide?
   a. muscular
   b. cardiovascular
   c. nervous
   d. integumentary
   e. none of the above

2. The lacrimal ducts empty into the
   a. nose
   b. mouth
   c. throat
   d. trachea
   e. none of the above

3. The nasal septum is made of
   a. epithelial tissue
   b. tendons
   c. bone
   d. cartilage
   e. none of the above

4. Which of the following is NOT a function of the vestibules?
   a. warm incoming air
   b. smell
   c. filter air
   d. help create speech sounds
   e. none of the above

5. Olfactory receptors are located in the
   a. superior meatus
   b. middle meatus
   c. inferior meatus
   d. oropharynx
   e. none of the above

6. Microorganisms that enter with air and are filtered out are destroyed by
   a. cilia
   b. mucus
   c. enzymes and acid
   d. hairs
   e. none of the above

7. The pharynx is divided into how many portions?
   a. 2
   b. 3
   c. 4
   d. 5
   e. none of the above

8. Which portion of the pharynx connects with the esophagus?
    a. eustachian tube
    b. oropharynx
    c. nasopharynx
    d. laryngopharynx
    e. none of the above

9. Which of the following is NOT one of the single pieces of cartilage in the larynx?
    a. arytenoid
    b. thyroid
    c. cricoid
    d. epiglottis
    e. none of the above

10. Which of the following cartilages is rod shaped?
    a. cricoid
    b. arytenoid
    c. corniculate
    d. thyroid
    e. none of the above

11. Together with the epiglottis, which of the following helps to keep food or liquids from entering the larynx?
    a. corniculate cartilage
    b. cuneiform cartilage
    c. vestibular folds
    d. vocal folds
    e. none of the above

12. Which of the following structures function as resonating chambers?
    a. pharynx
    b. mouth
    c. nasal cavities
    d. paranasal sinuses
    e. all of the above

13. Where does the trachea divide into left and right primary bronchi?
    a. cricoid cartilage
    b. fifth thoracic vertebra
    c. arytenoid cartilage
    d. fifth cervical vertebra
    e. none of the above

14. If the C-shaped incomplete rings of cartilage in the trachea were complete closed rings, what could you not do?
    a. breathe
    b. eat
    c. swallow
    d. talk
    e. none of the above

15. If a foreign object gets by the trachea, it would most likely get caught in the
    a. right primary bronchus
    b. left primary bronchus
    c. secondary bronchi
    d. tertiary bronchi
    e. none of the above

16. Which of the bronchi are segmented?
    a. right primary
    b. left primary
    c. secondary
    d. tertiary
    e. none of the above

17. The lungs are
    a. rod shaped
    b. wedge shaped
    c. leaf shaped
    d. cone shaped
    e. none of the above

18. The right lung has how many lobes?
    a. 1
    b. 2
    c. 3
    d. 4
    e. none of the above

19. The left lung has how many lobes?
    a. 1
    b. 2
    c. 3
    d. 4
    e. none of the above

20. Which does a lobule NOT contain?
    a. lymphatic vessel
    b. a venule
    c. an arteriole
    d. bronchioles
    e. none of the above

21. Atria are found in the
    a. bronchopulmonary segment
    b. alveolar ducts
    c. alveoli
    d. segmented bronchi
    e. none of the above

22. The third process of respiration is
    a. inhalation
    b. external respiration
    c. internal respiration
    d. exhalation
    e. none of the above

23. Destruction of the walls of the alveoli occurs in which disease?
    a. emphysema
    b. bronchitis
    c. cystic fibrosis
    d. pulmonary fibrosis
    e. none of the above

24. The disease common in infants is
    a. emphysema
    b. pulmonary fibrosis
    c. hyaline membrane disease
    d. pertussis
    e. none of the above

25. Which of the following is an inherited disease?
    a. cystic fibrosis
    b. pulmonary fibrosis
    c. hyaline membrane disease
    d. pertussis
    e. none of the above

CHAPTER 18   THE URINARY SYSTEM

CHAPTER OBJECTIVES

After studying this chapter, you should be able to:

1. Define the function of the urinary system.
2. Name the external layers of the kidney.
3. Define the following internal parts of the kidneys: *cortex, medulla, medullary pyramids, renal papillae, renal columns,* and *major* and *minor calyces*.
4. Name the parts of a nephron, and describe the flow of urine throughout this renal tubule.
5. List the functions of the nephrons.
6. Explain how urine flows down the ureters.
7. Describe micturition and the role of stretch receptors in the bladder.
8. Compare the length and course of the male urethra to the female urethra.
9. Name the normal constituents of urine.

ACTIVITIES

A. COMPLETION

Fill in the blank spaces with the correct term.

1. The urinary system consists of two _____, two _____, one _____ and one _____.

2. The kidneys are crucial in maintaining _____.

3. If kidney failure occurs, medical treatment consists of _____.

4. The elimination of wastes by the kidneys is called _____.

5. The kidneys regulate the concentration of _____ in body fluids and blood.

6. The regulation of hydrogen ions is _____ regulation.

7. The enzyme renin helps regulate _____ _____.

8. The liver, the skin and the kidneys all participate in the synthesis of _____.

9. The ureter leaves the kidney through the _____.

10. There are _____ layers of tissue surrounding each kidney.

11. The smooth, transparent, fibrous connective tissue membrane connecting with the outermost covering of the ureter is the _____ _____.

12. The mass of fatty tissue is the _____ _____.

13. The tips of the cortex are the _____ _____.

14. The cortex and the renal columns make up the _____ of the kidney.

15. The minor calyces collect _____.

16. Urine leaves the kidney through the _____.

17. The nephrons are the _____ units of the kidney.

18. The innermost layer of Bowman's glomerular capsule is made up of cells called _____.

19. The endothelial-capsular membrane is the site of _____ _____ and _____ _____ from the blood.

20. The part of Henle that is highly permeable to water and solutes is the _____ _____.

21. The kidney is supplied with blood from the left and right _____ _____.

22. About _____ of blood passes through the kidneys every minute.

23. The interlobar arteries are found in the _____ _____.

24. The nerve supply to the kidney comes from the _____ _____.

25. The process that transports substances out of the tubular fluid and back into the blood is _____ _____.

26. The bladder wall has three layers of smooth muscle known as the _____ muscle.

27. Micturition is precipitated by _____ _____.

28. Urine in the urethra is transported by _____.

29. _____ is caused by a high concentration of uric acid in the plasma.

30. _____ is an inflammation of the urinary bladder.

B. MATCHING

Match the term on the right with the definition on the left.

31. _____ helps adjust filtration pressure

32. _____ kidney cavity

33. _____ inner layer around the kidney

34. _____ outer layer around the kidney

35. _____ striated triangular structure

36. _____ point toward the kidney center

37. _____ cortex and renal pyramids

38. _____ collecting funnel

39. _____ double-walled globe

40. _____ Bowman's capsule and glomerulus

41. _____ U-shaped structure

42. _____ capillary network in the kidney

43. _____ smooth muscle in the bladder wall

44. _____ caused by uric acid in plasma

45. _____ helps regulate urine production

a. parenchyma

b. Bowman's capsule

c. glomerulus

d. renal corpuscle

e. loop of Henle

f. detrusor muscle

g. gout

h. aldosterone

i. renal pyramids

j. renal papillae

k. renal sinus

l. renin

m. renal pelvis

n. renal capsule

o. renal fascia

C. KEY TERMS

Use the text to look up the following terms. Write the definition or explanation.

46. Adipose capsule: _____

_____

47. Arcuate arteries: _____

_____

48. Bowman's glomerular capsule: _____

_____

49. Cortex: _____

_____

50. Descending limb of Henle: _____

_____

51. Detrusor muscle: _____

_____

52. Distal convoluted tubule: _____

_____

53. Endothelial-capsular membrane: _____

_____

54. Erythropoietin: _____

_____

55. Glomerulus: _____

_____

56. Interlobular arteries: _____

_____

57. Internal urinary sphincter: _____

_____

58. Left renal artery: _____

_____

59. Left renal vein: _____

_____

60. Loop of Henle: _____

_____

61. Major calyces: _____

_____

62. Nephrons: _____

_____

63. Papillary ducts: _____

_____

64. Parenchyma: _____

_____

65. Peritubular capillaries: _____

_____

66. Renal capsule: _____

_____

67. Renal columns: _____

_____

68. Renal papillae: _____

_____

69. Renal plexus: _____

_____

70. Renal pyramids: _____

_____

71. Renin: _____

_____

72. Trigone: _____

_____

73. Ureter: _____

_____

74. Urethra: _____

_____

75. Urine: _____

_____

D. LABELING EXERCISE

76. Label the parts of the urinary system as indicated in Figure 18-1.

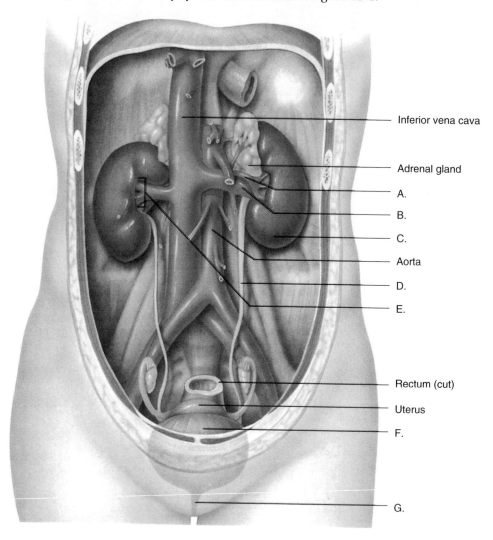

Inferior vena cava

Adrenal gland

A.

B.

C.

Aorta

D.

E.

Rectum (cut)

Uterus

F.

G.

a. _____

b. _____

c. _____

d. _____

e. _____

f. _____

g. _____

77. Label the parts of the kidney as indicated in Figure 18-2.

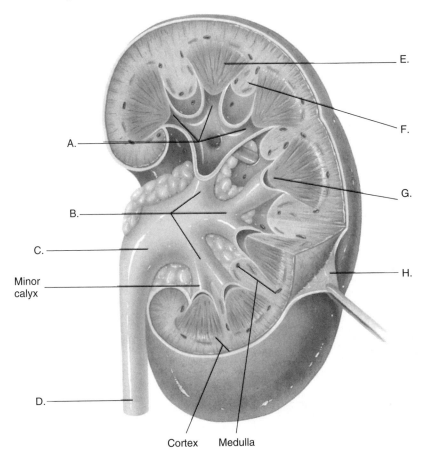

E.

F.

A.

G.

B.

C.

H.

Minor
calyx

D.

Cortex   Medulla

a. _____

b. _____

c. _____

d. _____

e. _____

f. _____

g. _____

h. _____

E. COLORING EXERCISE

78. Using Figure 18-3, color the proximal convoluted tubule, the distal convoluted tubule and the loop of Henle orange; the interlobar artery and the afferent arteriole red; the interlobar vein blue and the collecting duct yellow.

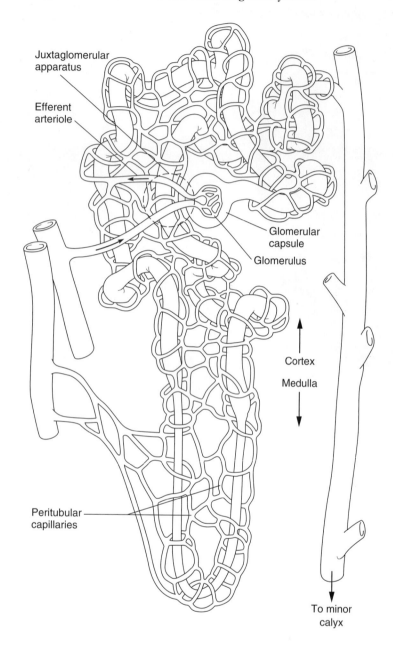

Juxtaglomerular apparatus

Efferent arteriole

Glomerular capsule

Glomerulus

Cortex

Medulla

Peritubular capillaries

To minor calyx

F. CRITICAL THINKING

Answer the following questions in complete sentences.

79. How do the kidneys help to maintain homeostasis?

80. How do the kidneys compensate for excessive perspiration?

81. Explain the part the kidneys play in the regulation of erythrocyte concentration.

82. Describe the role of the kidneys in teeth and bone development.

83. Why isn't hemodialysis a perfect substitute for kidney function?

84. Explain renal calculi and their treatment.

85. How does the endocrine system aid the kidneys to maintain homeostasis?

86. Explain why it can be said that the effects of aging on the urinary system begin as early as age 20.

87. Differentiate between a urologist and a nephrologist.

G. CROSSWORD PUZZLE

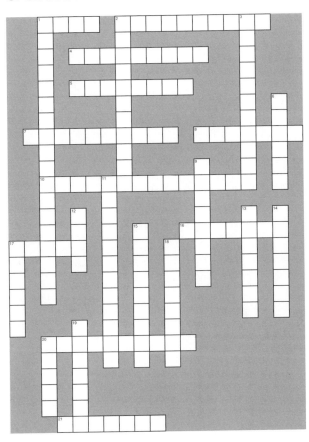

Complete the crossword puzzle using the following clues.

ACROSS

1. High uric acid in plasma

2. Cortex and renal pyramids

4. Waste elimination

5. Urinary bladder inflammation

7. Capillary network surrounded by podocytes

8. Transports urine by peristalsis

10. Stimulates red blood cell production

16. Veins connecting to interlobar veins

DOWN

1. Kidney inflammation

2. Capillaries form interlobar vein

3. Voiding

6. Outer kidney area

9. Functional units of kidneys

11. Procedure which filters blood

12. Transformed from ammonia by liver

13. Kidney stones

14. Inner kidney area

ACROSS

17. Formed by three processes in nephrons

20. Active vitamin D

21. Smooth triangular region of bladder

DOWN

15. Visceral layer of Bowman's capsule

17. Transports urine to the bladder

18. Three layers of bladder wall smooth muscle

19. Stores urine

20. Collects urine from renal pyramids

CHAPTER QUIZ

1. A scant amount of urine is called
   a. hematuria
   b. polyuria
   c. oliguria
   d. pyuria
   e. none of the above

2. Pus in the urine is called
   a. hematuria
   b. polyuria
   c. oliguria
   d. pyuria
   e. none of the above

3. Urine in the blood is called
   a. hematuria
   b. polyuria
   c. oliguria
   d. pyuria
   e. none of the above

4. Hemodialysis is the same as
   a. hematuria
   b. polyuria
   c. oliguria
   d. pyuria
   e. none of the above

5. Besides the urinary system, which system controls urine production and micturition?
   a. muscular
   b. endocrine
   c. nervous
   d. integumentary
   e. none of the above

6. Which system besides the urinary system is involved in the production of vitamin D?
   a. muscular
   b. endocrine
   c. nervous
   d. integumentary
   e. none of the above

7. Urea is the product of the liver breaking down
   a. water
   b. ammonia
   c. sugar
   d. starch
   e. none of the above

8. Which of the following is NOT one of the processes used by the nephrons in forming urine?
   a. glomerular filtration
   b. micturition
   c. tubular reabsorption
   d. tubular secretion
   e. none of the above

9. How much of the kidney can be nonfunctional and still keep the person alive?
   a. $\frac{2}{3}$
   b. $\frac{1}{2}$
   c. $\frac{1}{3}$
   d. $\frac{3}{4}$
   e. none of the above

10. The regulation of pH is the control of which ions?
   a. hydrogen
   b. potassium
   c. calcium
   d. sodium
   e. none of the above

11. The active form of vitamin D is
   a. calcium
   b. calciferol
   c. chloride
   d. sodium
   e. none of the above

12. The innermost layer of the kidney is the
   a. renal sinus
   b. hilum
   c. renal capsule
   d. renal fascia
   e. none of the above

13. The part of the kidney consisting of connective tissue and fat is the
    a. renal sinus
    b. hilum
    c. renal capsule
    d. renal fascia
    e. none of the above

14. The part of the kidney that anchors it is the
    a. renal sinus
    b. hilum
    c. renal capsule
    d. renal fascia
    e. none of the above

15. The millions of microscopic collecting tubules make up the
    a. nephron
    b. parenchyma
    c. pyramids
    d. cortex
    e. none of the above

16. In the ducts of the pyramids, urine is directly collected by the
    a. nephrons
    b. minor calyces
    c. major calyces
    d. ureter
    e. none of the above

17. Podocytes make up which layer of Bowman's glomerular capsule?
    a. visceral
    b. parietal
    c. outer
    d. cortex
    e. none of the above

18. The visceral layer of Bowman's capsule and the endothelial capillary network make up a(n)
    a. vein
    b. capsule
    c. endothelial-capsular membrane
    d. tubule
    e. none of the above

19. The papillary ducts empty into the
    a. renal capsule
    b. renal pelvis
    c. renal fascia
    d. pyramids
    e. none of the above

20. Those materials in the blood responsible for the acid or alkaline components of the blood are
    a. salts
    b. sugars
    c. electrolytes
    d. plasma
    e. none of the above

21. The renal artery divides into several branches that enter the parenchyma. In the renal columns they are called
    a. interlobar arteries
    b. arcuate arteries
    c. interlobular arteries
    d. efferent arteries
    e. none of the above

22. Glomerular capillaries unite and form the
    a. interlobar arteries
    b. arcuate arteries
    c. interlobular arteries
    d. efferent arteries
    e. none of the above

23. The peritubular capillaries form the
    a. arcuate vein
    b. interlobular vein
    c. interlobar vein
    d. efferent vein
    e. none of the above

24. The kidney's nerve supply comes from the
    a. central nervous system
    b. peripheral nervous system
    c. parasympathetic system
    d. sympathetic system
    e. none of the above

25. All of the following are part of the process of urine formation EXCEPT
    a. tubular formation
    b. glomerular filtration
    c. tubular reabsorption
    d. tubular secretion
    e. none of the above

26. Increased blood pressure is a result of
    a. tubular formation
    b. glomerular filtration
    c. tubular reabsorption
    d. tubular secretion
    e. none of the above

27. The daily production of urine depends on all of the following EXCEPT
    a. fluid intake
    b. temperature
    c. humidity
    d. emotional state
    e. none of the above

28. The detrusor muscle consists of how many layers?
    a. 1
    b. 2
    c. 3
    d. 4
    e. none of the above

29. The stretch receptors in the bladder begin to send messages when there is how much urine in the bladder?
    a. 700–800 mL
    b. 500–600 mL
    c. 400–600 mL
    d. 200–400 mL
    e. none of the above

30. Which of the following can become acute following strep throat?
    a. cystitis
    b. gout
    c. glomerulonephritis
    d. glycosuria
    e. none of the above

CHAPTER 19   THE REPRODUCTIVE SYSTEM

CHAPTER OBJECTIVES

After studying this chapter, you should be able to:

1. Name the internal parts of the testis.
2. Explain the effects of testosterone on the male body.
3. Describe the process of spermatogenesis.
4. Follow the path of a sperm from the seminiferous tubules to the outside.
5. Define *semen* and what glands contribute to its composition.
6. Name the three parts of the male urethra.
7. Describe the development of a follicle before and after ovulation.
8. Describe the process of oogenesis.
9. Name the parts of the uterus.
10. Name the external genitalia of the female.
11. Describe the phases of the menstrual cycle.
12. Describe lactation and the function of the mammary glands.
13. Name the phases of labor.

ACTIVITIES

A. COMPLETION

Fill in the blank spaces with the correct term.

1. Cell division resulting in 23 chromosomes in the egg and sperm is called _____.

2. Immediately following the union of sperm and egg, the fertilized egg is designated a _____.

3. When producing sperm, the testes are considered _____ glands.

4. When the testes are producing the hormone testosterone, they are _____ glands.

5. The testes are raised and lowered in reaction to changes in _____.

6. The inside of the scrotum has _____ sacs; these sacs are separated by a _____.

7. The _____ _____ extends inward and divides the testes into small compartments called lobules.

8. In the testicular lobules are found the _____ _____.

9. Meiosis occurs in the _____ _____.

10. Sertoli cells provide _____ for the sperm, and the interstitial cells of Leydig produce _____.

11. The acrosome contains _____, which help the sperm penetrate the ovum.

12. Mitochondria provide energy for the _____ of the sperm, which propels it on its journey.

13. The straight tubules lead to the _____ _____.

14. The sperm leave the testes through the efferent ducts and enter the _____ _____.

15. The seminal duct is another name for the _____ _____.

16. The part of the urethra found in the penis is the _____ urethra.

17. Three sets of accessory glands add secretions to the semen. The ones contributing the most are the _____ _____.

18. Protection of the sperm against bacteria is the function of _____.

19. As exocrine glands, the ovaries produce _____, and as endocrine glands they produce _____ and _____.

20. The _____ of the ovary contains ovarian follicles.

21. An egg is an ovum and an immature egg is an _____.

22. After the egg is ejected from the follicle, the follicle becomes the _____ _____.

23. The total number of eggs a woman can produce is determined at _____.

24. It is in the primary oocytes that _____ occurs.

25. It is the very small cell called the _____ _____ that is nonfunctional.

26. The funnel-shaped opening at the end of each fallopian tube is called the _____.

27. Fertilization takes place in the _____ _____.

28. The _____ _____ is the opening of the cervix into the vagina.

29. The visceral peritoneum of the uterus is a serous membrane known as the _____.

30. During the menstrual phase, a clear membrane called the _____ _____ develops around the eggs.

31. The ovum is not released directly into the uterine tube but into the _____ _____.

32. The beginning and end of the menstrual cycle in a woman's life are called _____ and _____.

33. The recess surrounding the vaginal attachment to the cervix is called the _____.

34. The mons pubis is also called the _____.

35. The _____ _____ of the external genitalia contain numerous sebaceous glands.

36. The glands homologous to the male Cowper's glands are the _____ glands.

37. The size of the breast is determined by the amount of _____ _____.

38. Human chorionic gonadotropin (HCG) is secreted by the _____ _____.

39. At the ninth week, the embryo is known as a _____.

40. _____ is the name given to childbirth.

B. MATCHING

Match the term on the right with the definition on the left.

41. _____ cellular division that produces sex cells

42. _____ elevates the testes

43. _____ connective tissue covering the testes

44. _____ daughter cells

45. _____ supply nutrients for sperm

46. _____ produced by the interstitial cells of Leydig

47. _____ where sperm cells mature

48. _____ secrete alkaline mucus

49. _____ penis head

50. _____ prepuce

51. _____ covers the surface of the ovary

52. _____ mature follicle with the mature egg

53. _____ white body

54. _____ transport eggs to the uterus

55. _____ between the body and cervix

56. _____ uterine middle layer

57. _____ yellow body

58. _____ external female genitalia

59. _____ veneris

60. _____ secrete and eject milk

a. fallopian tubes

b. Sertoli cells

c. myometrium

d. graafian follicle

e. foreskin

f. cremaster muscle

g. germinal epithelium

h. corpus luteum

i. corpus albicans

j. Cowper's glands

k. primary spermatocytes

l. vulva

m. epididymis

n. mons pubis

o. tunica albuginea

p. meiosis

q. lactation

r. glans penis

s. testosterone

t. isthmus

C. KEY TERMS

Use the text to look up the following words. Write the definition or explanation.

61. Acrosome: _____

_____

62. Areola: _____

_____

63. Chorionic vesicle: _____

_____

64. Chorionic villi: _____

_____

65. Clitoris: _____

_____

66. Corpus albicans: _____

_____

67. Corpus hemorrhagicum: _____

_____

68. Corpus luteum: _____

_____

69. Ectoderm: _____

_____

70. Efferent ducts: _____

_____

71. Ejaculatory duct: _____

_____

72. Endometrium: _____

_____

73. Fimbriae: _____

_____

74. Hymen: _____

_____

75. Internal os: _____

_____

76. Labia majora: _____

_____

77. Lactiferous ducts: _____

_____

78. Lesser vestibular/Skene's glands: _____

_____

79. Mammary glands: _____

_____

80. Menstrual cycle: _____

_____

81. Mesoderm: _____

_____

82. Oogenesis: _____

_____

83. Ovarian cycle: _____

_____

84. Ovarian follicles: _____

_____

85. Parturition: _____

_____

86. Perineum: _____

_____

87. Placenta: _____

_____

88. Progesterone: _____

_____

89. Raphe: _____

_____

90. Rete testis: _____

_____

91. Semen/seminal fluid: _____

_____

92. Spermatic cord: _____

_____

93. Spongy/cavernous urethra: _____

_____

94. Umbilical cord: _____

_____

95. Vagina: _____

_____

96. Vaginal orifice: _____

_____

97. Vasectomy: _____

_____

98. Vestibule: _____

_____

99. Vulva/pudendum: _____

_____

100. Zygote: _____

_____

D. LABELING EXERCISE

101.   Label the parts of the male reproductive system as indicated in Figure 19-1.

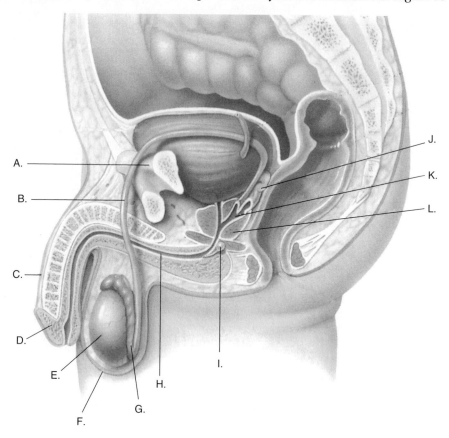

a. _____

b. _____

c. _____

d. _____

e. _____

f. _____

g. _____

h. _____

i. _____

j. _____

k. _____

l. _____

102. Label the parts of the female reproductive system as indicated in Figure 19-2.

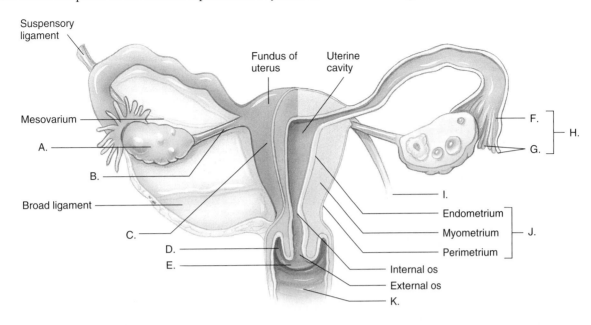

a. _____

b. _____

c. _____

d. _____

e. _____

f. _____

g. _____

h. _____

i. _____

j. _____

k. _____